Venus
&
Serena

SERVING FROM THE HIP

Ten Rules for Living, Loving, and Winning

with Hilary Beard

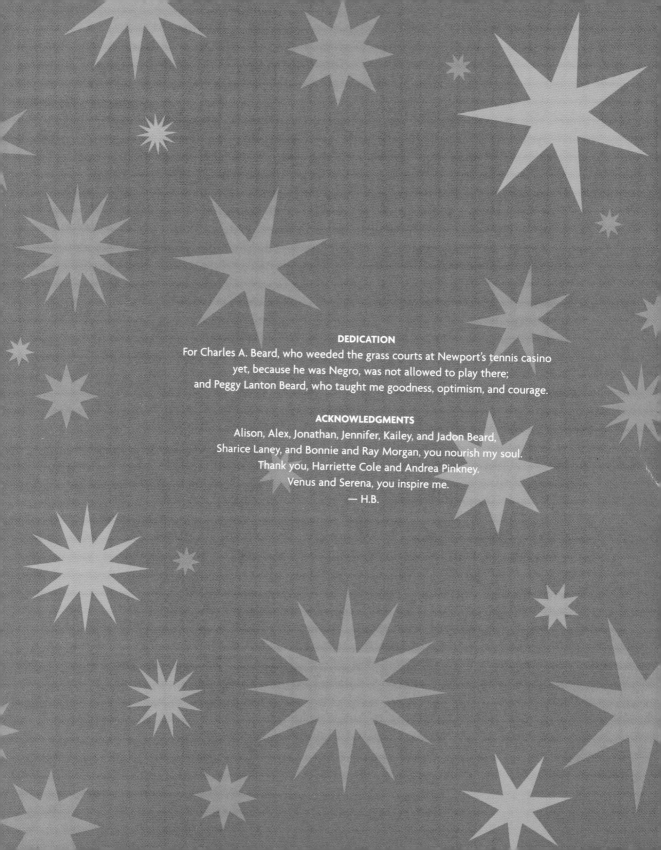

DEDICATION
For Charles A. Beard, who weeded the grass courts at Newport's tennis casino
yet, because he was Negro, was not allowed to play there;
and Peggy Lanton Beard, who taught me goodness, optimism, and courage.

ACKNOWLEDGMENTS
Alison, Alex, Jonathan, Jennifer, Kailey, and Jadon Beard,
Sharice Laney, and Bonnie and Ray Morgan, you nourish my soul.
Thank you, Harriette Cole and Andrea Pinkney.
Venus and Serena, you inspire me.
— H.B.

Venus & Serena

SERVING FROM THE HIP

Ten Rules for Living, Loving, and Winning

with Hilary Beard

HOUGHTON MIFFLIN COMPANY

BOSTON 2005

LIBRARY OF CONGRESS CATALOGING-IN-PUBLICATION DATA
Williams, Venus, 1980–
Venus and Serena : serving from the hip / by Venus and Serena Williams with Hilary Beard.
p. cm.
ISBN 0-618-57653-3
1. Williams, Venus, 1980– 2. Williams, Serena, 1981– 3. Tennis players—United States—Biography.
4. African American women tennis players—Biography. I. Williams, Serena, 1981– II. Beard, Hilary.
III. Title.
GV994.A1W55 2005
796.342'092'2—dc22
2004013204
ISBN-13: 978-0618-57653-1
Design by Sheila Smallwood and Georgia Rucker

Manufactured in the United States of America
RMT 10 9 8 7 6 5 4 3 2 1

CONTENTS

A WORD FROM
VENUS AND SERENA'S MOM

*W*henever I look into my mind's eye and think back on Venus's and Serena's lives, I'm just amazed at what they've accomplished. Growing up, they spent a great deal of time playing tennis, and I knew they would make it as professionals, but I never thought about the amount of success they would have—traveling all over the world, appearing on TV and in magazines, and all of the other incredible opportunities they experience daily. Back when I was pregnant with each of them, their father and I would get up every day at 5:30 a.m. to practice, because I wanted to be the best player I could be. After they were born, they practically lived and breathed tennis—Serena actually tottered around the court while she was still in her baby walker. In my wildest dreams I hoped they'd redefine the sport and make everyone else up their game. But I had no idea their lives would take off like *this!*

As their mother, I just knew there were certain things I wanted to teach them. The most important was to place God first in their lives and always follow His guidance. Venus and Serena do that, which is how I know that everything in their lives will always fall into place even though they make mistakes just like everybody else. I also encouraged them to always give their best effort. "If you work hard now, it will be easy later," I would tell them. But when it came to tennis, I balanced that advice by saying, "If anytime you feel like you want to quit, you can. You don't have to do this to be successful. Whatever you do, I'm proud of you." Still, they practiced day in and day out, even though many times I know they were tired. And I can't remember either of them ever complaining. I have to give them a lot of credit for being so dedicated. They were adults before I learned how much they loved rainy days so that they could take time off from practice.

I taught them to strive for excellence, not to gain acceptance from people—you'll

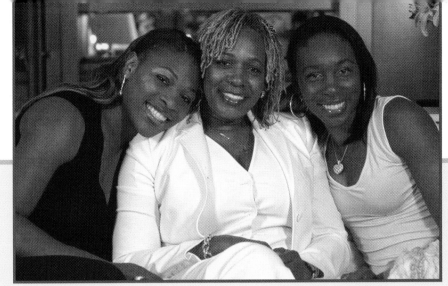

Venus and Serena with their mother, Oracene Price.

always feel disappointed if you look for recognition from others—but to satisfy themselves. "Life is to be enjoyed," I'd say. And loving yourself enough to do your best contributes to happiness. No matter what kind of work they chose to do in life, I wanted them to laugh, smile, and have fun, like Magic Johnson did on the basketball court. Thankfully, that is what happened. By the time they were eighteen, each of them had come to me about a year apart and said, "Thanks, Mom. I love my life." That's the most exhilarating statement any mother can hope to hear. Yes, now that they're rich, some things come easier, but Venus and Serena will be the first to tell you: Life is not about self or even material things; it's about caring and sharing with others.

I'm really grateful that my daughters have a good grasp on what living is all about. No matter what you do, you have a responsibility to others. "People are going to be watching you," I used to remind them. But I had no idea that Venus would one day tell me that she wanted to be a good role model and live a lifestyle that inspires others. Writing this book is one way of doing that. She and Serena give you the inside scoop on the values, beliefs, and behaviors that make their lives so fun and full of amazing options. They teach you ways of thinking and living that will allow you to feel in tune with God, confident of your abilities, strong in the face of adversity, and ready to create a dynamic future—no matter what exciting plans you have for your life.

Sweet dreams!

Oracene Price

WHY
WE WROTE THIS BOOK

As we travel all around the world to play in tennis tournaments, people ask us certain questions no matter where we go: *How have we become so successful? How do we deal with all of the criticism we receive? And how do we stay so close to each other even though we compete on the tennis court?*

From what our parents taught us while we were growing up and from our experiences in the world of sports, we've developed values and ways of conducting ourselves that have allowed us to excel professionally and lead happy personal lives. We wanted to share these ideas in the hope that we can help others achieve their big dreams just as we have achieved ours. When you turn the page you'll start reading

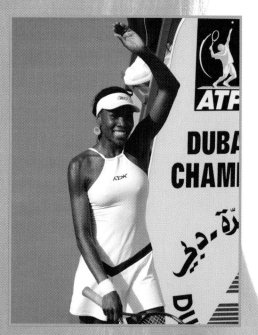

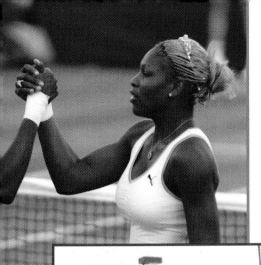

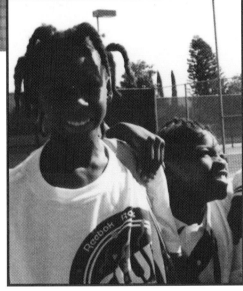

the first of ten chapters—one for each
of the Sister Rules—our code for living,
loving, learning, and playing with the
right crowd. Make these rules your
own as you go for your goals!

Sincerely yours,

Venus & Serena

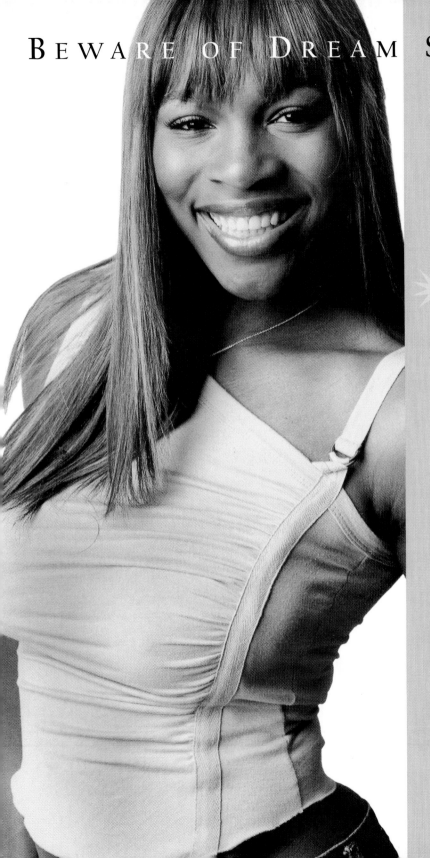

BEWARE OF DREAM STEALERS

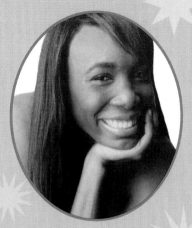

Sister Rule #1

I DON'T JUST DAYDREAM— I BUILD A DREAM TEAM. AND I DON'T LET OTHERS STEAL MY VISION.

SERENA

beware of dream stealers

Serena: We weren't always famous, we weren't always rich, and we weren't always the best players in the world. Not too long ago we were just two regular girls with very big dreams.

Venus and I spent our childhood in Compton, California, which is about twenty miles outside of downtown Los Angeles. A lot of people talk about Compton as a pretty tough place with drug dealers and gangs. But most of the people who live there work very hard to make ends meet. Our lives in Compton were normal, and we called it home. My mom was a nurse, my dad ran his own business, and we had three older sisters—Yetunde, Isha, and Lyndrea. Venus and I were a lot like the other kids our age, except that we had an unusual passion for a game called tennis.

Our father started our tennis dreams with a dream of his own. Before we were born he hoped that we would learn to play tennis and that maybe one day we could enjoy the big paydays he saw pros getting in tournaments on TV. So Daddy bought books and videos and taught himself and our mom how to play. Then when we were old enough, they taught us. Our other sisters played, too, but Yetunde and Lyndrea decided they didn't want to become tennis pros, and Isha got injured when she was playing in college. For some reason Venus and I really caught the tennis bug. And Daddy's dream became ours—we wanted to be the best players in the world.

"Our father was going around telling people we would be the best tennis players in the world."

Venus and I worked hard toward our goal from the very beginning. Dad and Mom would load us, our racquets, a broom, and a bunch of milk crates filled with old tennis balls into our old red and white Volkswagen van, and we'd head off to practice tennis. But unlike some families, we weren't going to a country club. We went to the local park, where grass grew in the cracks of the asphalt courts and there was so much broken glass and drug paraphernalia on the courts that we started each practice by sweeping them off. The conditions may not have been the best, but these courts became our second home. We practiced for several hours a day, most days a week, year in and year out, never losing sight of our dream.

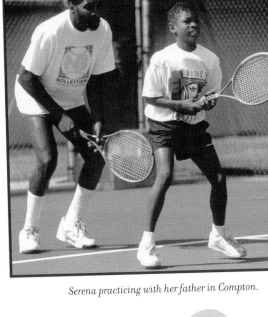

Serena practicing with her father in Compton.

Eventually Venus and I started to play in local tournaments to help us improve our skills. To many people's surprise, we earned number one rankings in Southern California's twelve-and-under (Venus) and ten-and-under (me) age groups. In the meantime, our father was going around telling people we would be the best tennis players in the world. He started calling Venus a "ghetto Cinderella." I'm sure a lot of people thought that he was crazy—and that we were, too. I mean, people were used to seeing tennis

"Our parents and our sisters shared the vision we had for our lives."

champions who were white. Who was ever going to believe that two black girls from Compton could become the best in the world? But we didn't stop playing, no matter how wacky our dream seemed to other people. Our entire family always had our backs. They were our Dream Team—the people who supported us day in and day out as we pursued our goals. Our parents and our sisters shared the vision we had for our lives and rallied together to help us. Even after they stopped playing, Yetunde, Isha, and Lyndrea spent countless hours patiently picking up hundreds of balls Venus and I hit when we practiced tennis drills.

Venus: Not long after we reached number one in our age groups, Mom and Dad made an unusual decision. They didn't allow us to play in any more junior tennis tournaments. They were starting to see that many of the young players were acting outrageous—cussing at adults and throwing their racquets—and getting burnt out by all the stress. Our parents didn't want that to happen to us. But a lot of people thought that withdrawing us from competition just didn't make sense.

When I was twelve and Serena was ten, our family moved to Florida, where we started to receive professional coaching. On top of

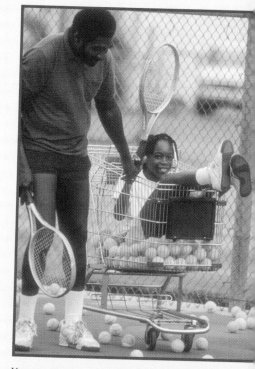

Venus getting a ride during practice with her father.

"To make it to the top, you have to stick to your goal no matter what."

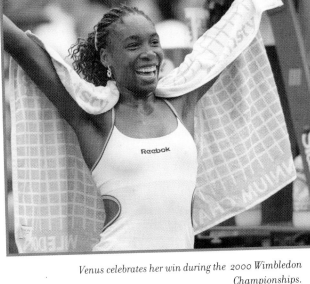

Venus celebrates her win during the 2000 Wimbledon Championships.

going to school, we practiced for six hours a day, six days a week. We still didn't play in junior tournaments, although most of our tennis peers did. But when I was fourteen, I played in my first professional competition. I won one match and then I got beat by the number one player in the world. But that didn't discourage me. Neither did my parents' decision that I wasn't allowed to play in many pro tournaments yet—not until I was a little older. Even though I was eager to compete more often, I trusted their judgment and just kept practicing. I stayed determined even though I was going to school and had to do my homework and help out at home. I was willing to work toward my dream every day, even when I didn't feel like it. Champions don't let anything stand in their way. To make it to the top, you have to stick to your goal no matter what.

Before long, Mom and Dad let me play in more pro tournaments. Within a couple of years I was moving toward the top of the rankings and closing in on my dream. At that point I set an additional goal for myself—to win Wimbledon, the prestigious tournament in London, England. Over the next couple of years, I played at Wimbledon on

"Dreams give you direction in life."

several occasions. But in 2000, when I turned twenty, I finally felt that my time had come. When I arrived at Wimbledon that year I felt like I had no choice but to win. I had been practicing very hard, I had been playing well, and I felt I deserved it. In fact, I was feeling *so* strong that I was just going to karate-chop anyone who got in my way. Unfortunately, that meant I had to beat Serena. But I was proud to achieve my goal even though it was at Serena's expense. Since then she's karate-chopped me back plenty of times. Later that year I won my first Olympic Gold Medal and I finally achieved my ultimate dream of being number one.

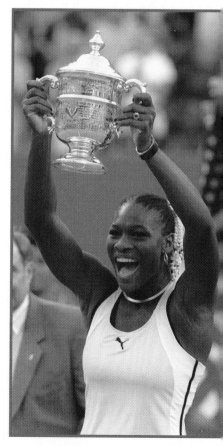

serena: **Venus and I** really like it when people tell us that they have big dreams. One of the most important things you can do for yourself is envision a fantastic future. Dreams give you direction in life. Everyone who is successful started with one.

Imagine what the world would be like without dreams. We wouldn't have many of the conveniences we enjoy if people didn't use their imaginations or weren't serious about making their desires come true. There would be no electricity or sliced bread or stoplights or television.

A victorious Serena at the 1999 U.S. Open.

"Venus and I are always thinking about our dreams."

Thank goodness for Martin Luther King, Jr.—he had a dream of equality for all human beings—otherwise, black people might still be fighting for our rights, and Venus and I wouldn't be able to play professional tennis. Venus and I are always thinking about our dreams. In fact, a famous African American poet named Langston Hughes wrote one of our favorite poems, "Dreams." We used to recite it often:

> Hold fast to dreams
> For if dreams die
> Life is a broken-winged bird
> That cannot fly.
>
> Hold fast to dreams
> For when dreams go
> Life is a barren field
> Frozen with snow.

Serena and I are lucky. The environment we grew up in was very pro-dream. Our parents protected us from the negative attitudes of people who didn't believe in us—Dream Stealers who tried to undermine our efforts. (To get the real deal on Dream Stealers, take the quiz on page 48.)

> ## "To become really great at something, you have to repeat it over and over so you can really ace it."

Unfortunately, a lot of people think that all you need to make dreams come true is good luck or a "big break." Having good luck always helps, but most times it takes a lot more than that—especially if you fantasize about becoming a superstar. You have to break big dreams down into very small steps then take them one at a time. To give you an example, before Venus and I ever played in a tennis tournament, we had to learn and perfect our shots. That means we practiced hitting thousands of forehands, thousands of backhands, and thousands of serves, day in and day out, long before anyone had ever heard of us or we had played in a single tournament. That's because to become really great at something, you have to repeat it over and over so you can really ace it. If you want to make the tennis team, you have to drill until you can almost hit shots in your sleep. If you want to get straight A's, you have to pay attention in class, ask questions, and do your homework every single day. If you want to be a singer, you need to do your vocal exercises over and over. If you have a great singing voice but would rather watch videos than practice, you'll never make it as a vocalist. You're better off choosing another dream. You have to sing because you love to sing, not because you want to be a star. Trust me—there will be many times when you'll have to practice your scales while your friends are out at the movies.

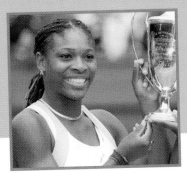

"When you're really going for something, you can't think about your doubts."

The more you practice, the better you get, and eventually you can move on to the next step—playing in local tournaments, participating in the science fair, singing in a recital, auditioning for a play, applying to a special program, or whatever. When you've mastered that level, you can move on to the next. But you have to excel at the fundamentals before you take the next step. Set a goal of perfecting your game, craft, or lessons no matter what you do.

In 1999, when I achieved my dream of winning the U.S. Open, I was certain I was going to win before the tournament even started. I deeply believed that my time had come. I had practiced hard for years. I had mastered all of my strokes. I had worked on being mentally tough. And I had prepared myself for my matches by studying my opponents. Beginning weeks before the tournament, I told myself over and over and over, "I'm going to win. I'm going to win." By the time I got to the championship match, I was absolutely, positively convinced. No doubts seeped into my mind at all. When you're really going for something, you can't think about your doubts. You have to push them out of your head and replace them with positive thoughts like "I can do this."

Sometimes dreams can be intimidating. Now that I've achieved my dream of becoming the number one female tennis player in the world, I've started to set goals for other areas of my life.

"When I first started thinking about designing my own fashion line, I felt a little insecure, but when I took the same steps to succeed in fashion as I took in tennis, I felt more confident."

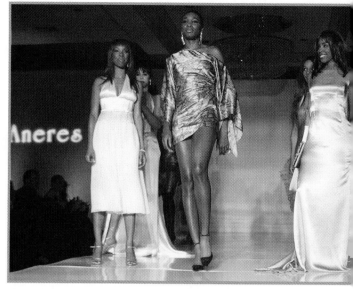

Venus, along with friends Kelly Rowland and Brandy, models one of Serena's designs during an Aneres fashion show.

Right now I'd like to design thirty or forty pieces of clothing and see them modeled on a New York runway. Although I'm very confident about tennis, when I first started thinking about designing my own fashion line, I felt a little insecure. A lot of other celebrities were coming out with their own brands, and I wondered if my clothes would be good enough.

But then I thought, "Why not?" They have their styles and I have mine. I'm going to put the same passion into my line of clothes—"Aneres" (that's Serena spelled backward)—that I put into my tennis. I'm going to keep developing my skills and do something toward my clothing line every day. I'm going to look for the people who can help me and invite them to be on my fashion Dream Team. When I thought about it like that—that I would take the same steps to succeed in fashion as I took in tennis—I felt more confident that I could make it.

"Along your journey—who knows?—you may make your wildest dreams come true!"

venus: The slick thing about working toward your goals is that even if you don't make it all the way, you will learn a lot about yourself and the world around you. When I was twelve I had this fun dream—I loved the rap group Kris Kross! I really wanted to meet them. A few years later I wanted to meet the rock band Green Day. Though I never met either group, listening to them taught me how much I love all kinds of music. I started playing the guitar, a hobby that I enjoy today.

As you pursue a dream, you may discover that you're not interested in it after all. That's perfectly fine. Singing may not be as fun as it looks on TV when you have to practice for hours on end. Instead, you may learn that you really like dancing. Dancing may expose you to choreography, which may be your true calling. As long as you are doing your best, learning and developing your talents, you're not wasting your time when you experiment with new activities. Along your journey—who knows?— you may make your wildest dreams come true!

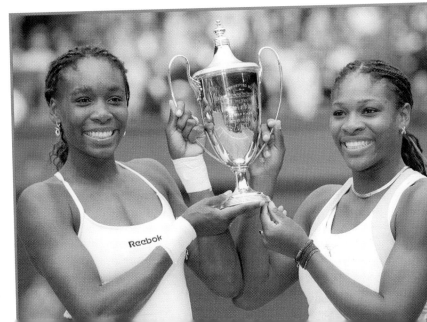

Doubles champs at Wimbledon 2000.

HOW TO CREATE YOUR
"DREAM TEAM"

*W*hatever you envision for yourself—becoming great at a sport, getting into a certain high school or college, performing in a play—you're going to need to build a support system—a "Dream Team"—of people who will help you achieve your goals. You can set yours in motion with a few easy steps.

1. **Get your parents in your corner.** Tell them about what you want to accomplish and ask them to help. If they don't agree with your goal at first, find out why. They may have good reasons for wanting you to do something else—like not wanting your grades to suffer or keeping you out of trouble. If that's the case, ask them what you need to do to get them on your side. Then work with them—show them that you can keep your grades up and that you have good judgment.

2. **Involve other adults.** In the same way that you involved your parents, invite your grandmother, an uncle, your favorite teacher, a school counselor, a youth leader at church, your coach, or your librarian to help. In addition to your parents (or if it can't be your parents), you want grownups on your team who are willing to talk about your ideas and problems.

3. **Build knowledge.** Ask all the members of your Dream Team if they—or someone they know—can help you learn more about your goal. Maybe you want to go to a certain school and your teacher knows someone who went there. Ask her if she'll introduce you to that person so you can learn about the school. Does anyone know a coach for the sport you like? If you like looking at pictures in magazines, can someone introduce you to a photographer who will let you visit his or her studio?

4. Dial the digits. When someone gives you the name of a person to contact—call that person! Don't let being scared, shy about what to say, or too busy get in the way of hooking up with someone who could help you.

5. Take advantage of every opportunity you get. If your uncle offers to read over the essay you need to write to get admitted to a special program, school, or college, send it to him with plenty of time for him to read it and get back to you with suggestions. If you want to be a doctor, tell your doctor. She may invite you to visit her office for part of a day to see what she does. Ask someone on your Dream Team to drive you there or help you map out the bus route so you arrive fifteen minutes early. Talk to your parents about the best day to go and ask them to help you pick out the appropriate clothes to wear.

6. Remember how important your best friends can be. You want friends who are supportive of the time you spend with your racquet, keyboard, or books. Your friends are on your Dream Team when they respect what you're trying to do.

7. Show appreciation. Send thank-you notes or e-mails to anyone you meet or visit. Tell your Dream Team how much you appreciate their support—often! They'll stick with you if they know you value their time and attention.

8. Be your own biggest fan. There will be rough spots when even the people who love you may temporarily lose faith. That's when you have to maintain your focus and believe in and root for yourself. In the end, no matter who is or isn't by your side, it's up to you to create the positive environment you need to nurture your dreams. No one can make **your** dreams come true but you.

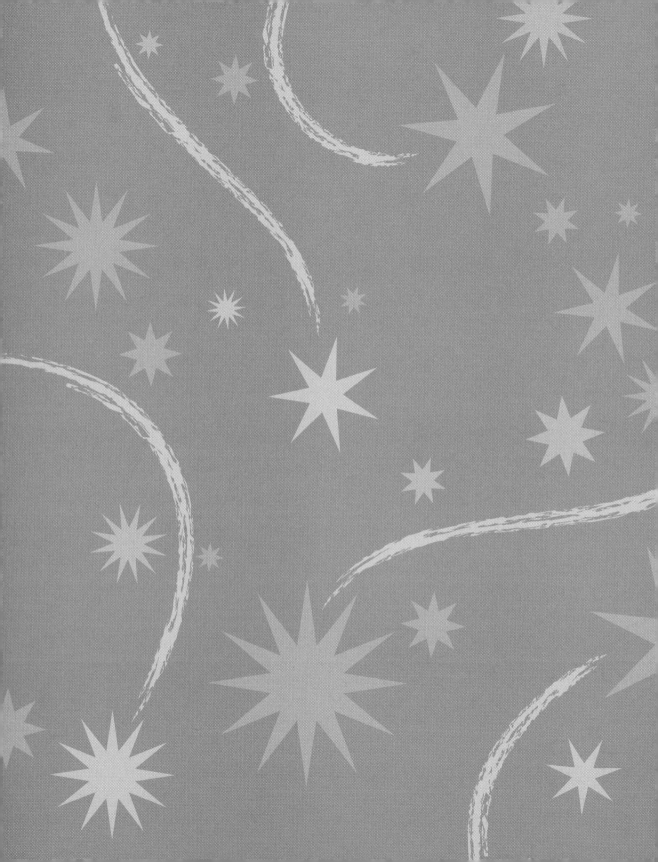

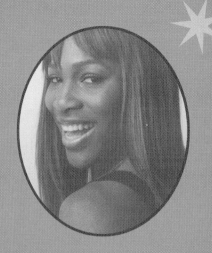

Sister Rule #2

WANT TO GET AHEAD? BOOK SMARTS GET YOU LIFE SMARTS.

VENUS

why school is cool

*V*enus: **Serena and I both graduated from high** school with higher than a B average. Our parents didn't allow us to come home with C's, which was fine with us, since we like to be excellent at everything we do. (There were times when I was bitter because I came home with a B.) Mom and Dad had high standards and always expected us to do our best. They taught us to put God first in our lives, our family second, education third, and our career after that. As the leaders of our Dream Team, they knew that even though our goal was to play tennis professionally, a racquet and a ball could take us only so far. We would need thinking skills to get ahead. Serena and I listened closely. And even though we were known to pass notes and throw a spitball or two, we stayed on top of our schoolwork and always tried hard. As a result, we also earned special privileges—like practicing tennis for hours each day. And because they didn't have to nag us to do well, our parents could relax and were fun to be around. Doing well in school helped make everybody happy!

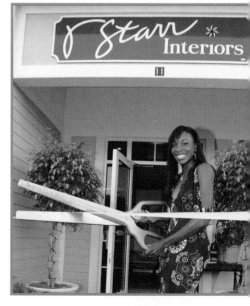

Venus cuts the ribbon to open V Starr Interiors. / ©TPL

"Serena and I go to college for the same reason that everyone else does—so that we have more options in life."

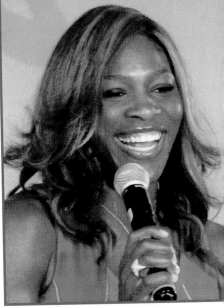

These days, even though we play tennis full-time, Serena and I also go to college. We usually try to schedule our classes during the fall because our travel schedule causes us to miss too many days if we try to go during peak tournament season, which is earlier in the year. Now, I know you're probably wondering why we even bother with college. You may be saying, "Why do you keep going to school when you're rich and don't have to?" Serena and I go to college for the same reason that everyone else does—so that we have more options in life. There *is* life after tennis, you know, and we *don't* plan to be sitting on the sidelines. Serena is developing her clothing line, Aneres, and dreams of her clothes being modeled in a fashion show in New York. To make her dream come true, she has a lot of preparing to do. She has to educate herself about design, business, marketing, and more. That's why she's starting while she's still playing tennis. I have an interior design company, V Starr Interiors, and I also want to create clothing. There are all sorts of interesting things that I want—and need—to learn in school. When my tennis career ends, I want to be like my older sister Isha. Isha has more degrees than anyone in our family. Because she's been in school for so much of her life, it seems like she must have ninety degrees by now. Actually, she has four, including a law degree and a master's in business administration—but it might as well be ninety since she is so well educated and has so many options in life.

Serena speaks about her new Nike clothing line at the Nike fashion show.

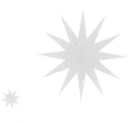

"When we're off the court, being well educated helps us handle our business dealings."

In addition to our formal education, we're constantly learning things on our own—foreign languages, for instance. We already speak French pretty well, so now we're also learning Spanish. This helps us to be more independent and allows us to talk with more people when we travel. On top of that, Serena is always perfecting her English. She just got through reading a book that taught her five hundred new vocabulary words. And I'm a big reader. I just *love* books. When I find a good one, especially about fashion, I pass it along to her.

serena: **Being well educated** helps us succeed both on and off the court. People watching us play tennis usually focus on the ball zooming around the court, how fast we run it down, or how hard we hit. But when you're the one playing, you know that there's more going on than what the crowd is able to see.

As Venus and I are chasing down balls and in the moments between points, our brains are always working. We are analyzing what's going on in the match. That means we're asking questions like *Is my opponent playing well today? What's her best shot? What's her weakness? How can I exploit it? When should I lay back and when should I move in*

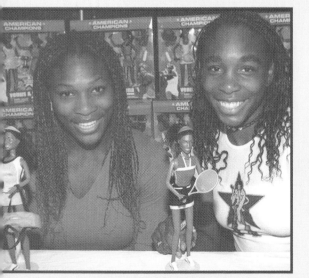

The Venus and Serena action figures debuted in 2000.

"Great thinking skills are essential to winning."

for the kill? We're also thinking about our own game: *What shot am I hitting best? How can I use that to my advantage? What isn't going well? How can I improve it?* We're asking ourselves all these questions and coming up with answers in the split second it takes for the ball to come rifling across the court. When the ball's being served at over ninety miles per hour from seventy-eight feet away, we have less than a second to move our bodies, decide *Where should I hit this?* and actually get the ball back. Even though people focus on our physical abilities, our minds must be sharp—not to mention quick. Great thinking skills are essential to winning.

When we're off the court, being well educated helps us handle our business dealings. From giving interviews to speaking at public appearances to negotiating endorsement contracts—we rely on skills we learned in English and math classes. And even though agents and advisors help us, having a good education allows us to be involved in all aspects of our careers. This is important, because many celebrities have been taken advantage of by people they trusted to manage their affairs. We don't want that to happen to us. Because we understand our business dealings, we don't have to give up all the control.

"Education will make such a positive difference in the quality of your life that you shouldn't sacrifice it for *anyone!*"

VENUS: **Serena and I were blessed** to really like school. But we also understand that not everyone does. Some kids have problems at home that make it hard to stay focused. Others get teased by their classmates, experience a learning challenge like dyslexia, or may even encounter a teacher who embarrasses them in front of the class. Even though these kinds of things happen, Serena and I believe there's nothing more important in life than getting a good education. We want you to become so determined to learn that you don't allow anyone or anything to come between you and your schoolwork—not your parents' personal problems, not teachers who don't care, or raggedy classrooms and books, not sports practice or big games, not being tempted by your boyfriend or girlfriend, not bullies, not a long bus or train ride, not the snow or wind or rain. Your parents' moods change, you'll have other teachers, teammates come and go, and so do boyfriends and girlfriends. Bullies flunk out, you get used to long rides on public transportation, and you can't control the weather. The people and conditions in your life change from day to day. But the things you learn will always stay with you. Knowledge is the one thing that no one can take away from you—ever, no matter what. This is really important for you to understand if you live in a place where the living and learning conditions are hard. The more you learn, the better your

"**There are lots of ways inside and outside the classroom for you to learn more and have lots of fun, too!**"

future will be and the more choices you'll have. Education will make such a positive difference in the quality of your life that you shouldn't sacrifice it for *anyone!*

If life's challenges make your school life tough, you need a Dream Team even more than the average person. Positive people can keep you motivated and focused on your goals when your environment is discouraging or you're feeling frustrated or even feel like quitting. So stay after school one day and talk to a teacher you like or who takes an interest in you. Tell her that you have big plans for your life and you want her to support you. Then do the same thing with other responsible adults and supportive members of your family. They can help you stay pumped up when other people around you aren't.

serena: **Not everyone learns best**—or finds classes that interest them—in a traditional school environment. I feel that way sometimes about my college education. Even though I like going to school a lot, I really *love* learning by doing. You can give Venus a book to read about fashion and she'll be happy studying all day. I like to read about fashion, too, but I'd much rather learn by rolling up my sleeves, drawing, checking out trends, and designing clothes.

"Should you give up? Of course not!"

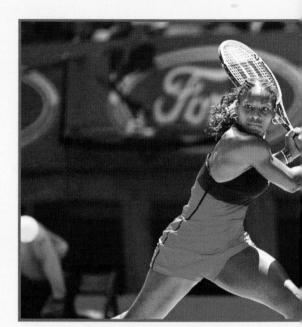

Serena focuses on the ball in a 2000 Australian Open match.

Still, I always work hard in my classes, because book smarts are always in style.

I think that everyone can benefit from hands-on experience. Say, for instance, you love animals and no classes or clubs in your school are even remotely related to them. Should you give up? Of course not! Ask the members of your Dream Team to help you put together a plan to obtain meaningful and fun educational experiences outside the classroom or in an untraditional manner. Maybe your counselor can help you get a job working or volunteering on weekends at the animal shelter. Maybe your mom can help you start a business feeding people's cats or walking dogs while they're on vacation. Maybe your dad can convince your scout troop to take a trip to an animal farm or local veterinarian's office. Or your school district has a special high school that teaches people about animals and plants and your favorite teacher can help you get into it. No matter what it is that you love to do, there are lots of ways inside and outside the classroom for you to learn more about it and have lots of fun, too. And

"Don't let others trick you into believing that being educated isn't cool."

there are always people who will love helping you do it. But you have to ask so they know what to offer.

Of course, it helps your case a lot when you have good grades. People are more willing to open doors for you, because your grades let them know that you're the kind of kid who will not waste their valuable time and effort. But even if your grades aren't the best, still be sure to ask. This may be just the motivation you need to get your schoolwork on track. And who knows? You may even get classroom credit for your outside activities. When Venus and I were in high school, we didn't have to take gym class because our school gave us credit for all the hours we spent practicing tennis! How's that for cool?

venus: **Unfortunately,** in some circles it's just not popular to be smart and do well in school. But if your acquaintances tell you that the things you're learning in class won't make a difference to your future, or if they tease you for being smart or studying hard, it's time to kick them to the curb. Take it from us: they don't know what they're talking about. Whether you want to be a doctor or a lawyer or an engineer or a singer or a rapper or a baseball player or an actor, being well educated is vital to your success. So don't let others trick you into believing that being educated isn't cool. Karate-chop those people out of your life and keep right on studying and learning! You have big plans for your future, and *now* is the time to prepare for it.

STUDY TIPS FOR ACES

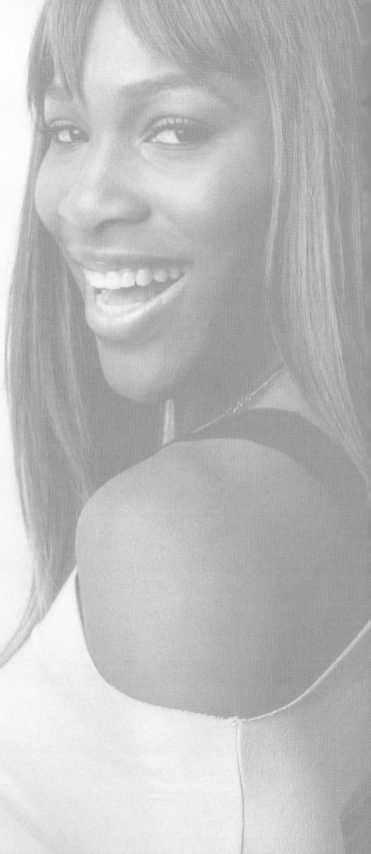

Doing well in school takes more than just being smart; you need to know how to study. These tricks of the trade help us get a lot of A's and B's.

1. Take notes. When we're in class, we write down the important points the teacher is saying. If she writes on the blackboard, we're sure to copy it down.

2. Do your homework. Things in your homework show up on quizzes and tests. We prepare ourselves by staying caught up. If we get behind, we stay after school and ask for help.

3. Start studying in school. When we have downtime between classes, we get our studying done. We don't use it to flirt with the cute guy on the other side of the room. Studying at school gives us more time for fun later.

4. Know your strengths. Should you study alone, with a friend, or in a study group? We change up by doing whatever works best for each subject.

5. Break it down. If our teacher tells us the test is on Friday, we figure out what we need to study in advance and review a little bit every day. That way, in the day or two before the test, we can ask the teacher things we don't understand. We don't wait until the last minute so we have to study the entire chapter in one night.

6. Take a break. We study in forty-five-minute increments and get up to stretch in between.

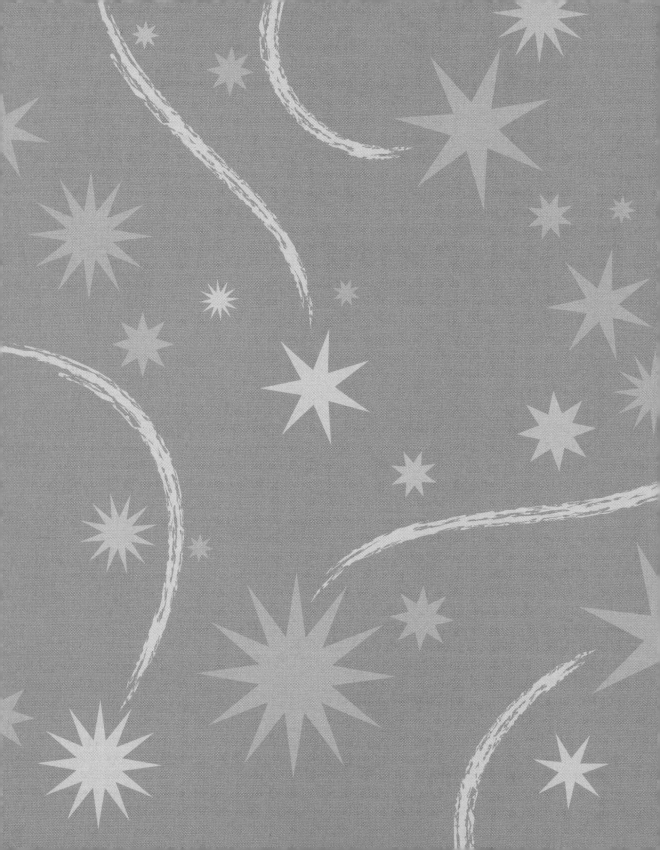

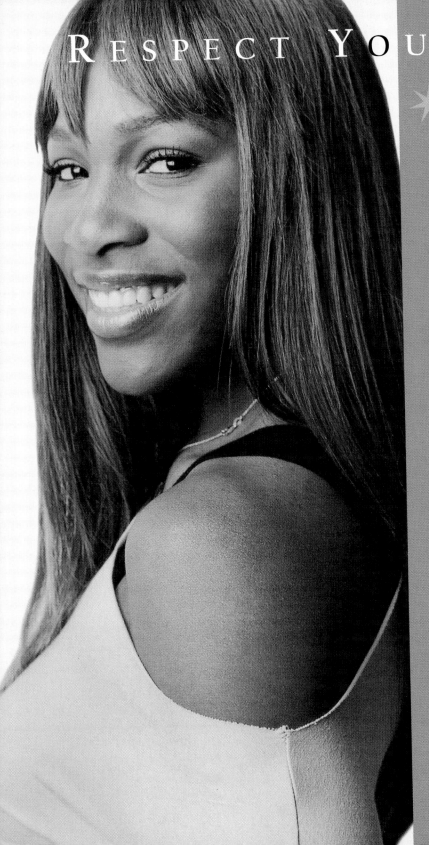

RESPECT YOURSELF

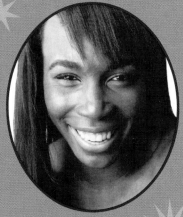

Sister Rule #3

Trophies don't tell whether I'm a winner. I win by doing right by me.

SERENA

Serena: Both winners and losers can be poor sports—whether they disrespect their opponents, treat their teammates and coaches badly, cheat, talk trash, or just straight up have a bad attitude. But knowing when to be a good sport about something and when to stand up for yourself can be tricky. There can be a fine line between being considerate toward others by giving them the benefit of the doubt and letting people take advantage of you. And while nobody wants to be known as a pushover, there are times when it's just best to walk away from a situation. When it's all over, you may still end up coming out on top, as I learned after I competed in the finals of the 2003 French Open.

I was playing an opponent from Belgium named Justine Henin-Hardenne. I had lost the first set, won the second, and was leading in the third. It was my turn to serve. Partway through the game, I tossed the ball into the air so I could serve it. That's when I saw Justine signal that she wasn't ready, so I intentionally knocked it into the net. I figured the umpire would have me play a "let"— a do-over—because in tennis that's the rule; if your opponent isn't ready, you replay the point. But it turned out that the umpire didn't see Justine signal me to stop, so he couldn't back me up. And when I had him ask her, well . . . let's just say that she didn't 'fess up. Now, we're all human and use bad judgment from time to time, and athletes all

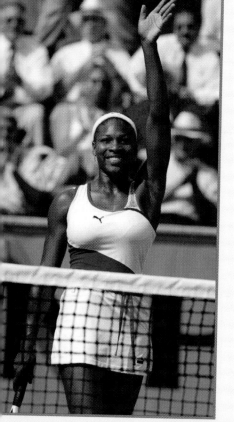

Serena waves to the crowd after her second-round win in the 2003 French Open.

"You earn your reputation by how you conduct yourself as much as from your talents."

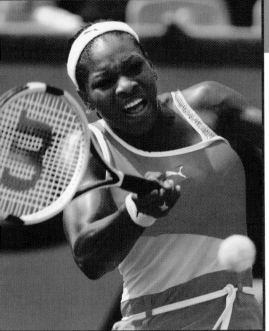

Serena in the 2003 French Open quarterfinals.

use a little gamesmanship—you know, when you do things to try to psych the other player out. But I thought this behavior crossed the line.

I stood up for myself by insisting to the umpire that I deserved to play a let. I wasn't about to roll over and let her take advantage of me. But there were two big problems: the ump didn't see Justine motion me to stop, so he couldn't side with me, and the match was being played in France. France is located next to Belgium, so Justine had "home-court advantage," so to speak. Her fans started to boo me—that *never* happens in tennis. In basketball and football crowds boo all the time and it's just considered part of the game. But tennis fans pride themselves on having "good manners."

I knew Justine had signaled, but I had no way to prove it. There's no instant replay in tennis. I was so mad at her for taking advantage of me that I wanted to chase her around the tennis court and swat her on the tush with my racquet! Fortunately, I remembered my parents' advice to always represent myself in

"Being a good sport and acting gracious sometimes takes you farther in life than winning."

a way I can feel proud of. So instead of continuing to complain to the umpire or practicing my forehand on her bottom, I decided to focus on winning the next point.

Unfortunately, I lost that point by blowing a shot. When that happened a lot of people in the crowd cheered my mistake. Then I lost the game. That made Justine's fans act even rowdier. For the first time in the match, I started feeling nervous. I tried to calm myself down and get my head together. But each time I messed up, the crowd jeered louder and louder. That is just *unheard of*. It would have been fine if they had stuck to cheering Justine's great shots. But by booing me and applauding my mistakes, the fans were really bad sports. I mean, imagine being surrounded by a stadium full of people who can't wait for you to flub something. Justine got psyched once the crowd got involved. She came from behind and beat me. *Ugh!* I *hate* when I let that happen.

After the match some reporters tried to get me to say negative things about Justine. But even though I was mad at her, I was more disappointed in my *own* performance. I had lost my composure on the court, but I wasn't going to make things worse by being a sore loser. *No* interviewer was going to talk me into saying something that I would regret later on but that they could turn into a headline. So I just told them that I was shocked that the crowd turned on me—which was true!—and I would just have to get tougher in case it happened again.

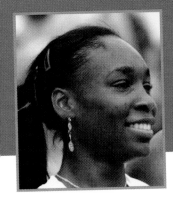

"There are times when it's just best to walk away from a situation."

Of course, I still had business with Justine, but I handled it woman to woman. (On TV you see people fighting in front of the camera. I think you get better results when you handle disagreements one on one and in private.)

But what happened next taught me a really important lesson. You know how people say "What goes around comes around"? Well, because television cameras caught Justine's actions on tape, not telling the truth made her look really bad. That caused her reputation with other players, fans, tennis officials, and members of the media to suffer. Lots of people told me that they felt bad about what happened. What started out as a bad situation for me became positive in the end. I learned that being a good sport and acting gracious sometimes takes you farther in life than winning.

Venus with her 2000 U.S. Open title trophy.

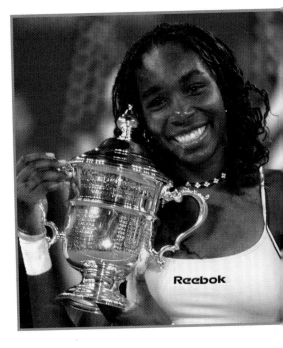

venus: I decided a long time ago

that no matter how many trophies I have at home, it's important to feel proud of how I handle myself. Whether you're a famous athlete or a regular person, you earn your reputation by how you conduct yourself as much as from your talents. I learned a lot from a controversial situation early in my career. When I was seventeen I competed at the U.S. Open for the first time. I was very excited to be there, but some of the players weren't very welcoming. In the semifinals I played against a

"Even bad situations offer us the chance to turn things around and make them turn out better."

twenty-three-year-old Romanian player named Irina Spirlea. Irina was ranked number seven in the world and I was number sixty-six, yet early in the week she had made negative comments about me. I ignored them, but when we met in the semifinals, I wanted to do my best on the tennis court!

The match was a tough one, and partway through we reached a point where we were to change ends of the court. Most of the time on a changeover, both players walk toward the side of the court that the umpire sits on, pass by each other, and head to their benches. But this time things didn't go quite that way. As Irina and I neared the net to cross over, the thought flashed through my mind that if one of us didn't step aside, we might run into each other. In that split second it dawned on me to engage in a little games-manship. I might be younger and new to the tour, I thought, but I'm going to let her know that her trash talking and mean attitude don't intimidate me. As we neared the net, I said to myself, "I'm not mov-ing." Well, she must have said the same thing inside her head, because the next thing I knew we were bumping into each other! I

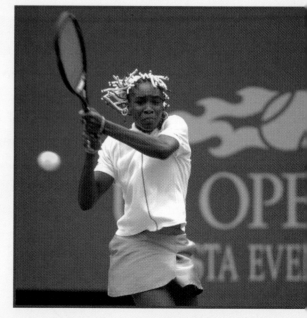

Venus playing in the 1997 U.S. Op

"Sometimes you get caught up in your emotions and can't foresee the possible consequences of your actions."

had assumed that she would step aside, and she probably thought I would, too. Sometimes you get caught up in your emotions and can't foresee the possible consequences of your actions.

I was surprised, but I stayed focused and kept my game face on. I walked to my bench, sat down, and studied the notes I had written to myself. By the time we headed onto the court to continue the match, I was so focused on winning, I had pretty much forgotten about the whole thing. I didn't give it much thought again until the press conference after the match. That's when I learned that reporters were making a big deal out of the incident. That's their job, you know—to get the scoop and create stories that will attract readers' attention. But it's my job to stay out of the headlines— unless they're about winning tennis matches. So when one of them asked me what had happened, I downplayed the whole thing and told them that I was just focused on winning the match. Another reporter informed me that while I was reading my notes, Irina was smirking and laughing and gesturing to her coach and friends in the stands. That was news to me since I had been focused on my notes and not on Irina. The reporter wanted me to comment, but I didn't have anything I wanted to say. The tennis world is a lot like being in school. If you say some-

"Make choices that keep the peace and make you feel proud of how you represent yourself."

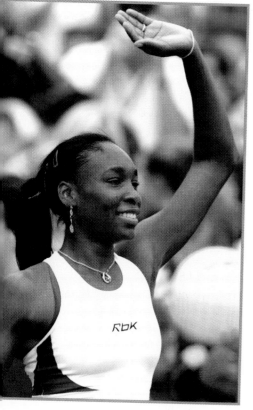

Venus after a victory at the 2002 U.S. Open.

thing bad about someone, they'll know about it within an hour. The best way to make something go away is to *keep your mouth shut!* But I guess Irina talked trash, because later on I read comments in the newspaper.

The unsportsmanlike things she said after the match turned the event into an international incident. In tennis it became known as "The Bump Heard 'Round the World." Since the match had been televised, our collision was replayed all over. So was the tape of her smirking about it. Acting smug made her look bad, even if her bumping into me wasn't on purpose.

I learned an important lesson. Initially, Irina and I engaged in the same behavior—we didn't get out of the other's way. But how we handled things afterward made a big difference in how people interpreted what happened and felt about us. I tried to minimize the incident. To tell the truth, once I realized that it was a big deal, I felt a little embarrassed. But Irina made the mistake of laughing and talking junk. That made her look as if she had run into me on purpose and—who knows?—maybe she did. It also made a lot of people feel that I was a "victim," even though I was also responsible for what happened.

"We all win some and lose some and make some mistakes — that's just the way the ball bounces."

serena: **The good thing is,** we can all learn from our experiences. We all go through times when we get caught in the heat of the moment. We let our emotions get the best of us, make silly mistakes, or may even lose our cool and act in an unsportsmanlike manner. But we can always get a hold of ourselves and keep things from getting worse. And as Venus's and my stories demonstrate, sometimes even bad situations offer us the chance to turn things around and make them turn out better. But that happens only when you make choices that keep the peace and make you feel proud of how you represent yourself.

The older you get, your attitude becomes more important. Being positive can help you get picked to do fun things— like being elected president of your class or captain of your sports team or leader of your youth group. Plus, you get special privileges from your parents because you're sending them the message that they can trust you. These experiences and opportunities will bring you closer to your dreams.

"If you handle things well the majority of the time,
you're going to be a winner in life—
on the court and off."

venus: But even though it's important to
act right, you don't want to let people run over you. When kids do things that
are mean, make you feel uncomfortable, or that don't fit with your values,
you have to learn when to make a racket. It's important to know when to use
phrases like: "Stop!" "That's enough." "I don't roll like that." "I won't play
by these rules." "I won't let you treat me that way." "Let's go talk to an adult
about it."

serena: Even though sometimes you
and your teammates—and maybe even your coaches and parents—get riled
up, nothing is so important that you should lose your self-respect, especially
not a game. We all win some and lose some and make some mistakes—that's
just the way the ball bounces. What is far more important is how you conduct
yourself. If you handle things well the majority of the time, you're going to
be a winner in life—on the court and off.

IT ISN'T COOL
TO LOSE YOUR COOL

Advice for keeping your head when other people have lost their minds—on or off the court.

1. Breathe. Sometimes when people get nervous, they forget to breathe. Taking several deep breaths can help you calm yourself.

2. Slow it down. Counting to ten or higher can help you regain your composure.

3. Play your game. When you're under pressure, it's not the time to try new things. Stick to what you know and the game plan you've been practicing. You'll feel more confident because it's familiar to you, and you're more likely to perform well.

4. Mind your business. You can't control what other people do or say. So stay out of the sideshow and focus on performing to your personal best.

5. Let go of the past. Instant replay is good for television, not for your mind. You can't fix plays that are already over. Rather than playing them over and over in your head, quickly figure out what you want to do differently, and prepare yourself for what's coming next.

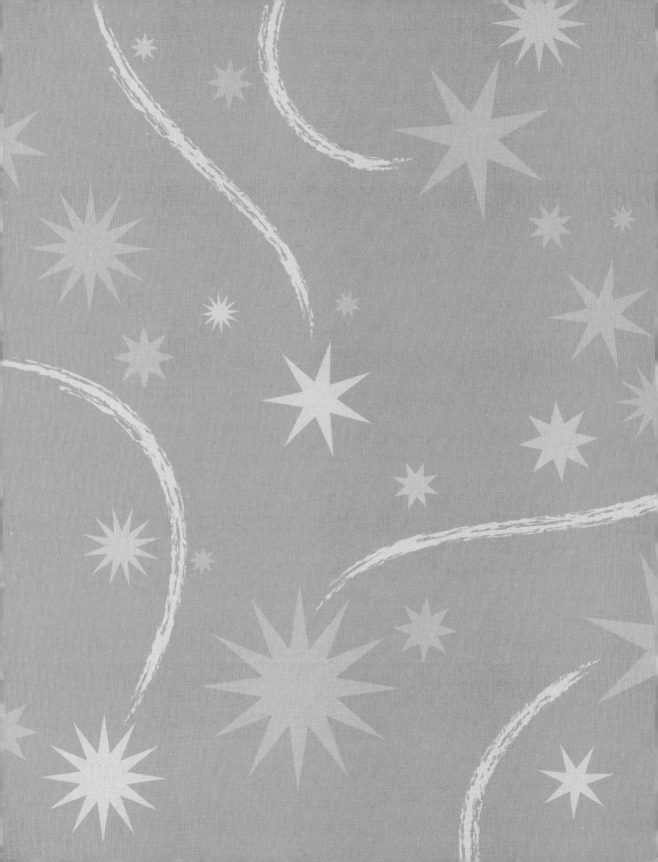

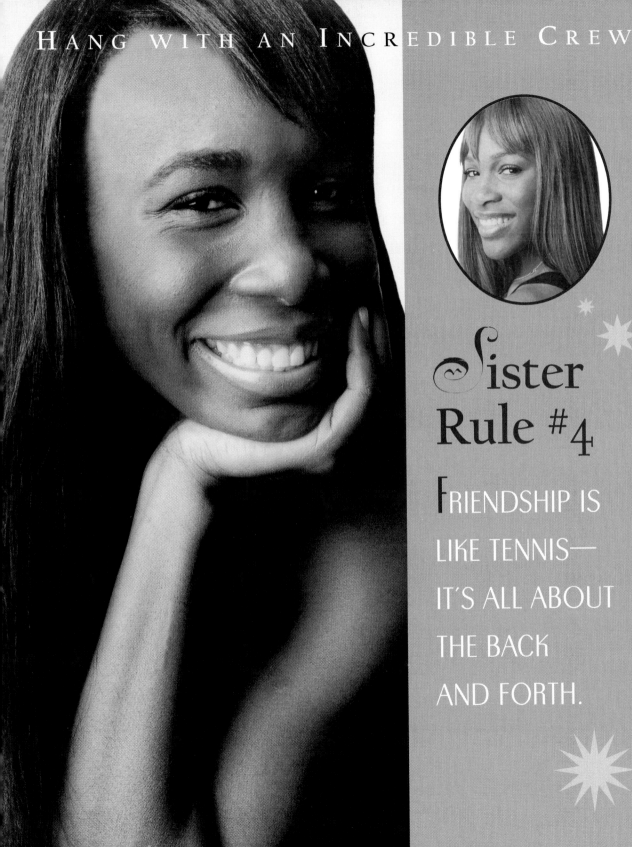

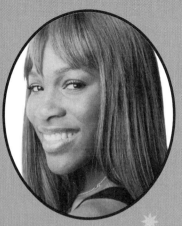

Sister Rule #4

FRIENDSHIP IS LIKE TENNIS— IT'S ALL ABOUT THE BACK AND FORTH.

VENUS

hang with an incredible crew

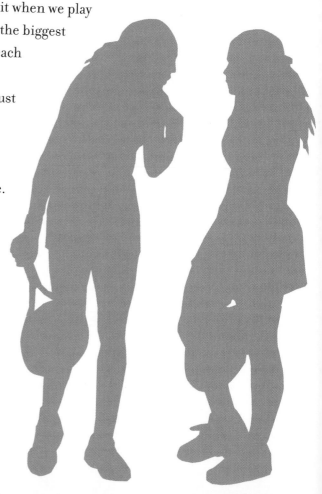

Venus: **In 1999 when Serena won the U.S. Open** before I had won any of the major tournaments, people seemed to think I was going to be devastated. I guess they assumed that jealousy would eat away at me and that our relationship would change for the worse. Apparently, they thought the same thing in 2002 when she became number one in the rankings. That year she defeated me in several Sister Slams—that's what the press calls it when we play against each other in the finals of the biggest tournaments—and I noticed that each time she beat me, certain people seemed to think my world would just fall apart.

I don't like to lose to anyone, including Serena—even in practice. And there are definitely times when I get mad at myself or feel disappointed in my performance. But to allow something as unimportant as a game ruin our friendship? *Puh-leez!* I come from a large family, and my sisters are my best friends. Whatever happens on the tennis court, it's not going to change my

"Nothing can keep me from celebrating when my best friend wins a match."

love for Serena or my pride in her accomplishments. I know better than anyone how much she's sacrificed to be a champion—how hard she's practiced, how many blisters she's gotten on her feet, how many parties and dates she's missed out on. No matter who wins or loses the tournament, anytime there's a Sister Slam it means we've been as successful as possible. Of course, everyone thinks it's cute that even when Serena beats me I sometimes pull out my camera and take pictures of her on the victory stand. But I'm not trying to be cute; I'm being serious. I want my own pictures of these events. Nothing can keep me from celebrating when my best friend wins a match.

serena: Venus and I

are really blessed. Long before fans and reporters knew us, our parents taught us that our relationship is much more important than being successful in tennis or getting ahead in the world. Our friendship with each other and our other sisters is one of the most important

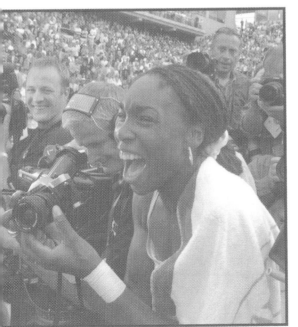

Venus takes pictures of her sister after losing to Serena in the 2002 French Open finals.

"Learn to distinguish between your true friends and people who are just acquaintances or associates."

and fun aspects of our lives. Venus and I know lots of people—tennis associates, schoolmates, friends from when we lived in California, fans—and we're always making new acquaintances. But we never forget that our parents, sisters, and closest friends are the people we can count on to have our best interests at heart. They are the people we entrust with our most personal thoughts, secrets, hopes, and heart's desires because, as true friends, they are honest and loyal. They help us nurture our dreams and make them come true. Of course, we support them, too.

Not everyone will have your back like that. That's why you can't let just any old person be your friend. Whether or not you're famous, it's important to learn to distinguish between your true friends and people who are just acquaintances or associates. Unfortunately, not everyone has your best interests at heart. As it says in the Bible, "Bad associations can spoil useful habits." That means not using good judgment in choosing your friends and hanging out with the wrong crowd can undermine all the good things you've done and great decisions you've made. Now that we're well known, Venus and I get approached by lots of people who claim to be our friends. They are often very pleasant people, but many times it turns out that they just want to borrow money. If we weren't able to tell the difference between the people who want something from us and our true friends, we would get scammed all the time. But even when you're not a celebrity, people have different reasons for wanting to be around you.

"I have found that it helps to restrict myself to hanging out with people who share my goals and values."

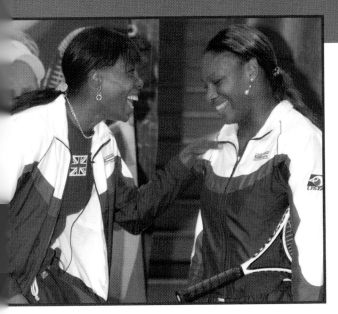

Sharing a laugh during a 2003 Fed Cup tennis clinic.

venus: **Serena**
knows a lot about friendship. She is very outgoing—much more than I am. Because of that she has a lot more friends than I do. I aspire to be like her. I admire how friendly she is and how easy it is for her to think of fun things to say to people she doesn't even know. I've always been kind of quiet and stayed to myself. But when I was a teenager, I would suddenly become popular whenever test time came around. The other kids knew that I studied hard and got good grades. They also knew that I didn't mind helping them out. So I would bail them out at test time, but I didn't fool myself into believing that they were true friends. It's not as if I had turned popular overnight or something. My classmates wanted to spend time with me because they needed my help. After the exam they would go about their business and so would I, until the next test came along.

In my life I have found that it helps to restrict myself to hanging out with people who share my goals and values. Lots of times people think about restrictions as being bad, especially when they're trying

"Your performance improves because there are inspiring people around you."

to get more privileges. It's true that some restrictions can reduce the amount of freedom you have—like being grounded. But there are also useful restrictions, ones that actually give you more choices in life because they protect you from negative influences and prepare you to be in the right place at the right time when exciting opportunities come along.

serena: **One restriction I put on myself** when I'm with my friends is that I try not to hang out real late at night. I'd rather go to sleep at a decent hour. That way I'm not dragging, exhausted, the next day and I have the energy I need to perform well on the court and in my other business dealings.

When you hang out with kids who are doing well, not only will you have fun, but you'll also benefit from something known as positive peer pressure. That's when your performance improves because there are inspiring people around you. If I had to motivate myself to train every day, sometimes I might decide to skip my workout and go to the movies. But since Venus is my true friend, she encourages me to train harder than I would if I were alone. Just being in her company encourages me, and playing tennis with her helps me elevate my game. Because she reads a lot and is always learning new things, she inspires me to keep up with my reading and educate myself.

One of my goals in life is to earn a college degree. But I wasn't planning to go to college at this point in my life—not while playing tennis full-time. Then one day Venus came home and told me she had signed me up for classes. I

"Playing tennis with Venus helps me elevate my game."

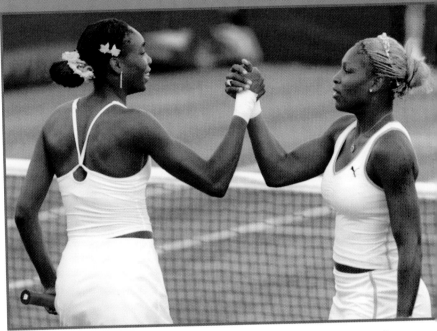

Celebrating a point during a 2002 Wimbledon doubles match.

couldn't believe it! And with my schedule, I had no idea how I could possibly get the work done. But she kept saying, "Come on, Serena, you'll love it. We'll be able to study fashion together. It will be a lot of fun!" So I gave in. "Why not?" I figured. That's what made me go ahead and start school now—a nudge from Venus. I never would have tried to attend college while playing tennis full-time, but I am really proud of these accomplishments and really appreciate Venus's encouragement.

venus: **You see how it works?** Serena is inspiring me to become more social . . .

serena: **And Venus motivates me** to educate myself more. That's the sign of a fabulous friendship!

THE REAL DEAL WITH DRUGS

Serena:

These days, all you have to do is turn on the TV and you can see people smoking weed or getting drunk in videos and on reality shows. They act like everyone does it and like it's a normal part of growing up. But trust me when I tell you that even though it may seem that way, not everyone gets high. I don't. And Venus doesn't, either.

Even though I'm known for tennis, I'm also involved in fashion and entertainment—industries a lot of people associate with drugs. I do my best to stay as far away from drugs as possible. One time I was at a Los Angeles Lakers game and ended up seated near someone who was intoxicated. Even though I really wanted to see the game, I got up and left before the second half started because I didn't want to be associated with someone who was high. Whenever I catch a whiff of weed, I immediately leave. It makes no sense for me to hang around trying to act cool, accidentally breathe some marijuana smoke, and get a positive result on a drug test. If I was in a car driven by someone I really didn't know well and we were pulled over and I learned that the driver was high, I would be considered guilty by association. My future is too important to jeopardize like that. And so is yours.

Hanging out with people who do drugs or drink alcohol—or, worse, getting high yourself—puts you in the middle of a bad scene. First of all, drugs and alcohol can damage your body and mind. There's no worse time to impair your thinking than during the time of your life when you're preparing for your future. And kids who get high look and act stupid—they have red eyes that are halfway closed and look horrible with any outfit, they laugh about dumb stuff, stagger around and bump into things, reek something awful, and to top it all off, sometimes they pass out or vomit. What's cool about that?

Plus, getting high has consequences—and not one of them is good. You can get in trouble with your parents, kicked off your sports team, expelled from school, busted by the police, or find yourself in the middle of a dangerous situation. Teens that get high or drink damage their relationships at home and with friends and shut down their opportunities in life. Some kids may think that it makes you hot stuff. But as our mother always told us: a lot of the kids who are the most popular in school don't make it very far in life.

WOULD YOU MAKE OUR TEAM?

Venus: There are times in every relationship when you have to decide where you stand—whether you're a Dream Teamer, Dream Stealer, or someone in between. Serena and I are very picky about who we associate with. Take this quiz to see if you would make the cut.

1. **Your best friend confides that she wants to try out for the school play, even though she's never acted before. What do you do?**
   a) Tell her to lose ten pounds and take acting lessons so she doesn't embarrass herself.
   b) Tell her it's a good idea but secretly hope she'll fail.
   c) Encourage her to go for it and offer to help her rehearse her lines.
   d) Joke about it on the bus, hoping that someone else will keep her from making a fool out of herself.
   e) Audition for the same part she does.

2. **Your volleyball team loses when a teammate makes a big mistake. What do you do?**
   a) Get mad and tell her it's all her fault.
   b) Pull her aside and say, "Don't sweat it—everyone has bad days."
   c) Gather the other players together and tell the coach to sit your teammate on the bench.
   d) Volunteer to come early and practice with her so she'll get her confidence back.
   e) B and D.

3. **You are shopping with your best friend when you both spot a fabulous outfit at exactly the same time. What do you do?**
   a) Rip it out of her hands and run to the dressing room to try it on.
   b) Tell her that you saw it first so you should be the one to buy it.
   c) Wait until she wears it to school and then criticize how it looks on her.
   d) Suggest that she try it on first, and if it doesn't fit or she doesn't like it, then you'll try it on.
   e) Tell her that it's not her style, hoping she'll leave it on the rack for you.

4. **Your girlfriend has a crush on a cute guy and is debating whether to let him know. What do you do?**
   a) Secretly tell him.
   b) Joke about it at the lunchroom table so he'll find out through the gossip grapevine.
   c) Get mad at her, figuring that if she has a boyfriend she won't hang out with you anymore.
   d) Start dressing nicer so that he'll notice you.
   e) Keep her secret and continue to focus on your studies.

ANSWERS

Question 1:

If you chose answer C, congratulations! Not only are you willing to encourage your friend—you're helping her achieve her dreams. If you act like this all the time, you could hang with us! Anyone who chose answer B gets props for being honest. It takes a lot of maturity to encourage your friend even though you may have mixed feelings about her succeeding. You did the right thing by keeping your negative thoughts to yourself while you work on becoming more positive. If you chose answers A or D, you may be a Dream Stealer—someone who steps on other people's dreams just because they don't have their own. Then again, you may know for a fact that your friend is a lousy actor. If so, figure out an incredibly tactful way to tell her while also encouraging her to shoot for the stars. That way you're building her up, not bringing her down. And if answer E was your choice, all we have to say to you is "tacky, tacky, tacky."

Question 2:

If you chose answers B or D, you're a really good friend. But an even better friend would do both—psych her up *and* help her get back on track, like Serena and I do for each other! Did you choose answers A or C? Read this chapter again, or you won't survive the cut for our Dream Team.

Question 3:

We just know you didn't choose answer A. If you did, re-read this chapter ten times! After you're done, read it one more time just to make sure the information sticks to you like Elmer's glue. Did you choose answer B, C, or E? We'd consider you an acquaintance, not a true friend, because you don't have your friend's best interest at heart. Answer D is the right choice. You could hang out with us!

Question 4:

The correct answer is E. It's always best to mind your business and keep your nose in your books. They are, after all, the reason you're in school in the first place. In our next chapter, we'll teach you to "Do You!"—to stay focused on what's important in your life and let everyone else handle what's important to them.

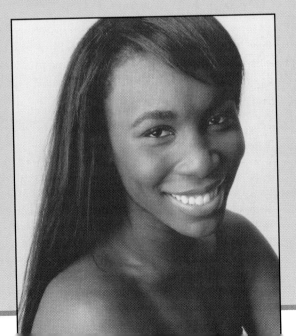

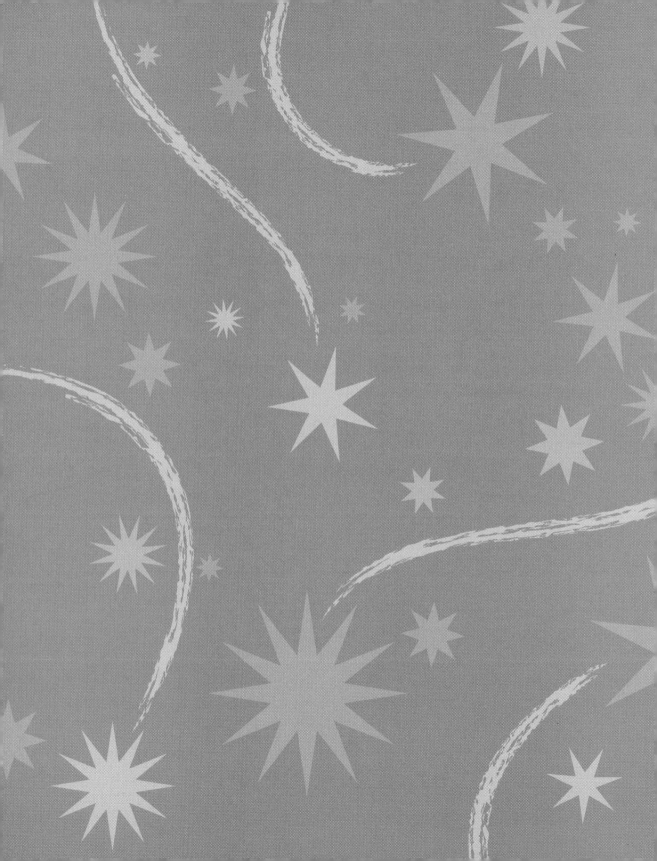

Be True—Do You

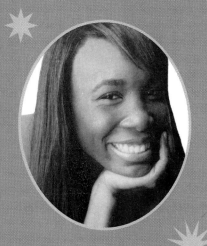

$\mathscr{S}$ister Rule #5

WHAT OTHERS THINK OF ME IS NONE OF MY BUSINESS. MY LIFE IS MY BUSINESS— PERIOD.

SERENA

Serena: **Back when we were** teenagers, before either of us had reached number one, a reporter asked Venus what her biggest dream was as a tennis player. She told him that she wanted to win Wimbledon. Later on another journalist asked me the same question. Since Venus had answered Wimbledon, I said Wimbledon, too. I figured that if Venus said it, it must have been a really cool answer. Afterward my father pulled me aside to talk about being myself. "You're your own person, Serena," he said. "You don't have to do everything Venus does." So the next time a reporter asked me about my dreams, I had an answer of my own. "I want to win the U.S. Open," I said. And in a few years, I did.

Because Venus and I are so close and I am her younger sister, I've always looked up to her. Until I was about eighteen years old, if Venus wanted to do something, I wanted to do it, too. If she liked it, I liked it. If she wanted to go somewhere, I was right behind her. And if I wasn't imitating her, I was copying one of my other sisters. Then I started to realize that life doesn't work that way. I had to make choices about who *I* wanted to be. Because if I did only the things Venus did, then I'd miss out on some of the things I really enjoy—like acting, which I love but Venus isn't that into. There can be only one Venus Willams, and the best person to play the part is Venus, of course. No one can do Venus better than Venus, and she can't do Serena better than me. My job is to focus on

> "Learning how to be true to myself was one of the most important things I have done in my life."

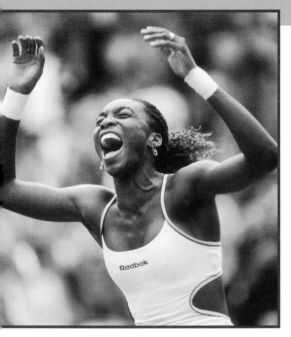

...yful Venus wins the 2000 Wimbledon Championship.

being the best Serena I can be—to do Serena—rather than worry about anybody else. That's one of the most important things I've learned in life. In fact, it's so important that I've turned it into a motto: Do You!

VENUS: **Learning how** to be true to myself was one of the most important things I have done in my life. This has involved taking the time to figure out what I think and how I feel about different issues and situations, and then having the courage to be honest with my family and friends.

Over the past few years, Serena and I have learned a lot about ourselves. And we're discovering how many ways we're different even though we're a lot alike. We're both always laughing and having fun. But Serena's more outgoing than I am, even though there are times when she's also shy. I'm more of an introvert, although I'm trying to become more outgoing. We both love to travel. But Serena loves Los Angeles, while I love New York and London and think L.A. is just okay. We both really like the guitar, but Serena prefers

"Sometimes I have to spend less time with friends and family so I can do what I love."

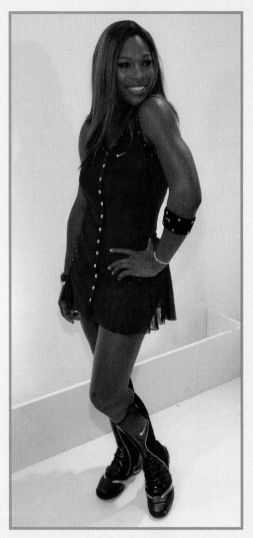

Serena introduces the Shox Boots from Nike's Serena Collection.

electric and I jam on the acoustic. Both of us are passionate about design. But she favors fashion and I like all types—art, fashion, jewelry, architecture, home décor. So even though we are a lot alike, these days sometimes we go separate ways to lead the lives we enjoy.

Making the adjustment to spending time apart from Serena has been the hardest part about knowing myself. But I've learned that sometimes I have to spend less time with friends and family so I can do what I love. At first it was a little scary. But now that I'm used to traveling on my own, I've learned that I really enjoy my own company. Even if I'm off in another part of the world, I never feel alone. They may be far away in distance, but my family never feels far from my heart. One time I was in between tournaments in Europe and I went to London and spent four days by myself. I really had a great time. I went around to antique markets, I saw the museum of London, I even went to Madame Tussaud's, a famous museum where they have life-size wax replicas of some of the most famous people in history. The figures look so real you'll swear you're standing next to a real person. Madame Tussaud's is my favorite museum!

> **"There's no need to be afraid of hanging out with yourself."**

Because I was by myself, I got to wander around at my own pace and look at and read about the people who were most interesting to me. I especially liked the chamber of horror, a really gruesome exhibit where they have wax mannequins of serial killers and the instruments that used to be used to torture people. It's kind of like being in a haunted house or watching a scary movie! I liked the dungeon and medieval areas much more than looking at the celebrities. And looking at kings and queens and Nelson Mandela was really, really fun. Now that I have spent that time on my own, I understand that it's important to have alone time. There's no need to be afraid of hanging out with yourself.

serena: These days, Venus and I talk on the phone and send text messages all the time, but we may not see each other for months. Following our own paths like this has been a big adjustment, but the sacrifice is definitely worth it. I would never have discovered a lot of amazing things about myself if I had followed her around for the rest of my life. And imagine if Venus and I had followed the advice of all the so-called "experts" who told us to only play tennis. We wouldn't be going to college, and there would be no V Starr Interiors, Aneres, acting, or other activities that bring us so much joy. I've learned to be selective in accepting advice. No one besides myself and members of my Dream Team are "experts" about my life. When I'm on the tennis court, I play by the rules of the game and keep the ball inside the lines. But my life is not a game.

"I've learned that no person outside of my Dream Team can be more of an 'expert' about my life than I am."

I determine my own goals and paint my own boundary lines. And I never, ever pay attention to people who want me to limit myself.

I feel *sooo* excited when I design new styles and get to see them on the runway. It's amazing how much more beautiful clothes look on a model instead of a mannequin. And then there's *acting!* Even though I feel awkward and nervous sometimes, making different characters believable is *really* interesting and challenging to me. Exploring these other interests occupies me so I don't miss my family as much, and tennis stays fun and my life always feels new and exciting. Now when Venus and I get together, there's much more to share and catch up on. And the most surprising thing has happened to me since I've started to do Serena. Instead of my always wanting to hang out with Venus, she claims that she's trying to hang out with me!

Venus: Because I am blessed to travel the world as I play tennis, I get exposed to different countries and cultures, which teaches me a lot about what I like and dislike. I've learned that I like all kinds of music—Indian and Arabic, for example. I always try to squeeze in a trip to an outdoor art market. And I'm willing to try any kind of food. One time when I was in Moscow, Russia, I ate in an Armenian restaurant one night, a Ukranian restaurant the next night, then a Russian restaurant, and a Georgian restaurant—just totally enjoying the experience. If anything, sampling different flavors from around the

"I get exposed to different countries and cultures, which teaches me a lot about what I like and dislike."

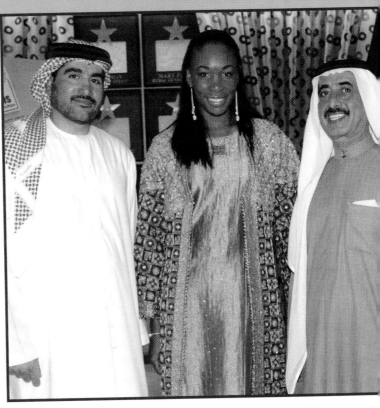

Venus wears a traditional Arabic dress in Dubai.

world makes me like American food a lot less. I prefer Thai food and Indian food and Japanese, Greek, and Middle Eastern to the food that we eat here. I wish I had time to cook. I'd like to try something exotic. I got a cookbook once that has international recipes, but haven't had a chance to use it yet.

And even though I don't have much time to sightsee while I travel for tournaments, I *have* had a chance to visit some pretty interesting sites. I went to the Grand Canyon when I was about six. And, of course, because I live in Florida, I've been to Disneyworld. I've also seen the Eiffel Tower in Paris, France; London Bridge in London, England (Remember the nursery rhyme? Well, there's really a London Bridge and it is still standing); the Sydney Opera House in Sydney, Australia; the Coliseum in Rome and Duomo cathedral in Florence, Italy; and the Kremlin and St. Basil's church in Moscow, Russia. (Look them up on the Internet.) I really liked St. Basil's. When you walk in one section, there are flowers painted on the ceiling and each flower is different. You feel like you're taking a step back in time. It's very, very cool!

"When I learn from my mistakes and figure out what I'd do differently, I discover important things about myself."

I also get to know myself by being human and making mistakes. I know this may sound crazy, but the errors I make can actually work to my advantage if I take the time to learn from them. To give you an example, if I could do it all over again, I would go to college earlier—right after graduating from high school. I think that waiting was a mistake, although I don't beat myself up for it. I hesitated at the time, but now I wish I had gone for it. If I had started earlier, I'd be much closer to graduating than I am right now. Because I work and go to school, graduating seems so far away—some days, almost farther than I can imagine. And I devoted so much of my life to tennis that I haven't learned about a lot of things that happen off the court. These days, I'm learning to manage my time better—to *make* time rather than complaining "I don't have enough." Instead of lounging in bed until nine in the morning, I get up early so I can do things like hop on the Internet to learn more about other careers. When I learn from my mistakes and figure out what I'd do differently, I discover important things about myself. The mistake helps me know what I *don't* want to do or be, which helps me become more focused.

serena: **You can even learn** a lot from getting in trouble. One time when I was nine, one of my girlfriends—let's call her Kimberly—had a crush on this boy we'll call Michael. For some reason I thought it would be funny if I forged love letters from Michael to Kim. The letters

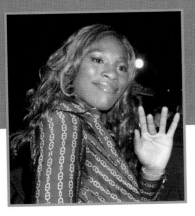

"I always try to treat people as I want them to treat me."

really embarrassed her. Eventually one of my friends didn't think it was funny anymore and told on me. The time had come to pay for my inconsiderate behavior.

I thought that nothing could be worse than seeing how angry Kim and Michael were at me when they found out what I had done. But I was also forced to spend the day standing in the principal's office in a "penalty box" where *everybody* could see me. The *entire school* found out what I had done to my friend. I guess you could say I got a dose of my own medicine. Getting punished publicly like that was very humiliating to me—probably as humiliating as it was for Michael to discover that I was writing fake love letters in his name or for Kimberly to learn that the love letters she was receiving weren't real after all. I learned a very powerful lesson that I carry forward with me in life: I will never intentionally embarrass anyone else again. And I always try to treat people as I want them to treat me.

venus: **As our lives** expose us to new people, places, experiences, and ideas, Serena and I try to make sure they're in line with both who we are now *and* who we want to be in the future. One way we do that is to stop to check in with our values. This works best for me when I carve out quiet time alone. The solitude gives me just enough space from other people that their

"We never, ever want to do anything that would embarrass our mom and dad."

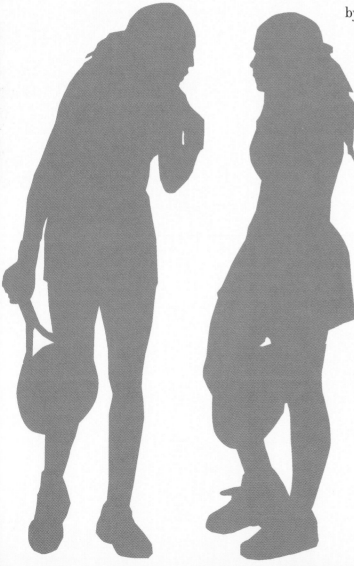

opinions don't influence me too much. (If I'm in a pinch and a situation is developing too fast for my comfort, I take a moment by ducking into the bathroom.) Also, we do a personal value check by reading the Bible every day. We travel with it everywhere we go and study and follow its guidance, like we did when we still lived with our parents. That way, when we're faced with situations that we're uncertain about, our relationship with God is always on our minds. Whenever I feel uncomfortable I ask myself, "What would God want me to do?" or "Would God want to see me doing this?" Serena and I also think about how our parents would feel about our behavior. We never, ever want to do anything that would embarrass our mom and dad. When we look at situations in these ways, the right choice is usually very clear.

serena: Once you
know what your life is about and your choices support your values, it's easier

"Not trying to be part of the 'in crowd' turned out to be in our best interests."

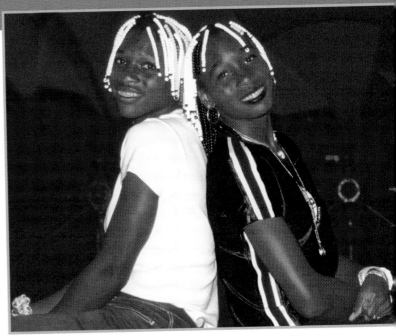

Serena and Venus in Australia, early in their professional tennis careers.

to stand up to peer pressure. When we were growing up, there was this group of kids who called themselves the Get-Along Gang. The kids in the Get-Along Gang were trying to be cute and cool. They cursed a lot, and you had to smoke to join their group. Everyone wanted to hang out with them. One day the head of the Get-Along Gang came to Venus and me and told us that we couldn't hang out with them. They said we weren't cool enough and we definitely weren't cute. At first I felt rejected. Then I thought about it for a moment. I realized, *"Hey!* I don't want to curse and smoke anyway. And my mom wouldn't like it if I got in trouble." I decided, "I don't even want to be in the Get-Along Gang. I can start my own group anytime I want."

Well, not trying to be part of the "in crowd" turned out to be in our best interests. Thank goodness our mother always told us not to worry about what other people think and that the people who are the most popular as teenagers don't always do well in life. Rather than smoking and getting in trouble, we followed her advice and focused on our dreams. We may not have been "good enough" then, but a lot of people think we're pretty cool now!

"I feel strong enough to remove myself from situations that don't make me happy."

venus: When I'm being true to myself, I feel strong enough to remove myself from situations that don't make me happy. One time, to satisfy a public relations commitment, I went to a party after a music awards show. Sometimes they can be a lot of fun. The food is fabulous, the music is great, and you get to meet your favorite music stars. But at this party a lot of people were smoking cigarettes—I hate the smell of cigarette smoke and it's so bad for my lungs! Then, while I was out on the dance floor, a girl next to me started dancing crazily. I don't know if she had been drinking or what, but I was about to move when she flicked her cigarette ashes all over me. Now, I was already feeling uncomfortable, but being turned into an ashtray really pushed me over the edge. I wanted to knock her upside the head with my purse! Fortunately for both of us I exercised self-control. But I had fulfilled my commitment to attend, and this party was definitely not for me. I told my crew, "I don't want to be a part of this scene." Then I left without them, since they wanted to stay.

"**Every day we have to decide whether to invest in our futures . . . or give in to the temptation to be irresponsible.**"

serena: **You would think** that now that we're adults and celebrities, our lives would be entirely different. But I can't help noticing how we get presented with a lot of the same choices and situations we experienced in junior high school. We're always meeting new people and have to decide who to make friends with and who to stay away from. We have a lot more freedom and have to figure out how to use it. And every day we have to decide whether to invest in our futures by studying, working hard, and saving money or give in to the temptation to be irresponsible.

Hasn't something like this happened to you or someone you know? Some weekends my friends want me to go to parties with them so I can get them into the VIP section. (That's the private area in a club where only celebrities and their friends can go. It helps us enjoy ourselves without having to sign autographs all night—which can be exhausting—or having people think we're mean if we aren't up to it.) Now, even though going dancing is a lot of fun, sometimes staying out late is not a

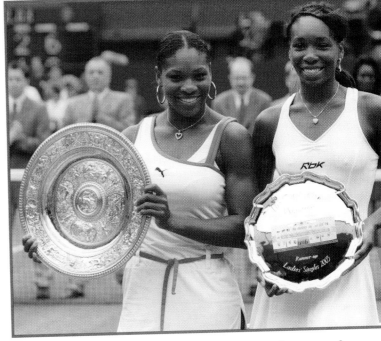

Standing together at the 2003 Wimbledon awards ceremony after Serena defeated her sister in the final.

"I live with the consequences of my choices."

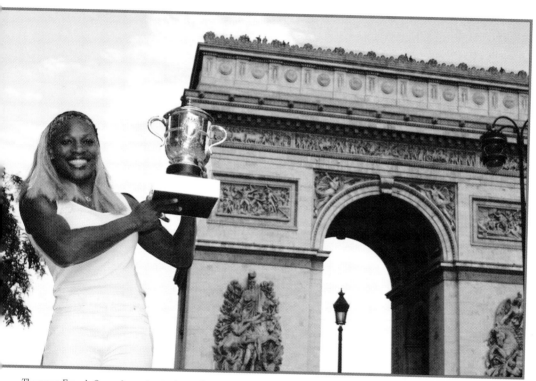

The 2002 French Open champion in front of the Arc de Triomphe in Paris.

good decision for me so I don't do it. I may need to get a good night's sleep and wake up early in the morning. Since *I* live with the consequences of my choices—no one else does!—I can't be trying to please other people. When *I* do what's right for *me*, I feel good about myself when other people are around and also when they're not. Sometimes it's worth it to stay home now so I have peace of mind later. I always know that another party will come around soon.

"Our goal is to make fantastic choices."

Because I always consider the consequences of the things I do, most times I make good choices. For instance, I don't waste a lot of time. Even though I don't read anywhere near as much as Venus does, my friends would tell you that I always have my nose in a book. I read French instruction books to keep my language skills sharp, since I don't know anyone who speaks French fluently. Sometimes my friends joke: "Serena is weird. She's always reading." But I don't care that they don't read. Our lives are different, and I do what I have to do to prepare myself. *I love languages!* When I go to the French Open I want to explore Paris and meet people and shop. Because I speak French and was taking Portuguese at one time, I understand Italian enough to get around because the languages are similar. I've also studied Spanish and German. Speaking many languages gives me the freedom to be myself and explore wherever I am in the world!

venus: **Being honest** means we have to make some tough decisions. Our goal is to make fantastic choices so that when the Williams sisters look in the mirror, Venus is happy with Venus and Serena is happy with Serena. Because we do that for ourselves, there's no one else we'd rather be!

GET TO KNOW
YOU

You don't have to travel to distant lands to figure out who you are. You can start exploring your world right in your own backyard. Did you know that treasure can be uncovered with just a pencil and notebook paper? Take quiet time alone and jot down the answers to the questions below. Share them with your parents or Dream Team and ask how they can help you make your deepest desires come true.

◆ If you could be any character on TV or in the movies, who would you be and why?

◆ If you could spend the day doing anything you wanted to, what would that be?

◆ If you could be anything you wanted to be, what career would you choose? How can you learn more about that line of work?

◆ What happened on the happiest day of your life, and why did it make you feel so good?

◆ List three things you would like to try that you've never experienced before. Then write down the first step you need to take to get closer to each one.

◆ What are you good at?

◆ What do other people tell you you're good at?

◆ What do you suspect you're good at but have never tried?

◆ What activity do you get so absorbed in that you lose track of time?

◆ If you could go anywhere in the world, where would that be and why?

◆ What kinds of activities do you daydream about?

◆ What do you enjoy doing that nobody knows about?

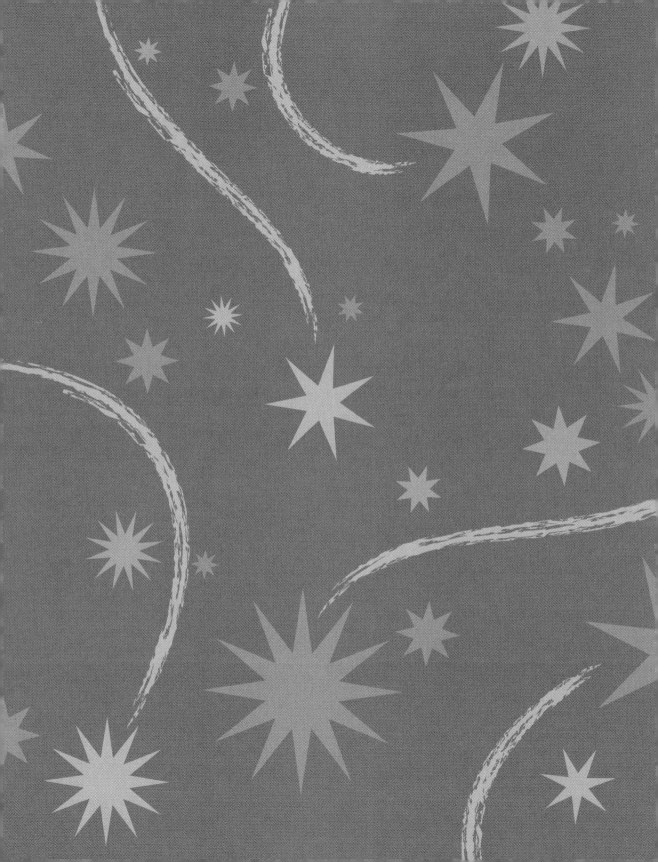

DON'T RUSH A CRUSH

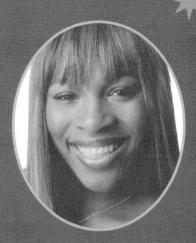

Sister Rule #6

BOYFRIENDS AND GIRLFRIENDS COME AND GO, BUT FRIENDSHIPS LAST FOREVER.

VENUS

don't rush a crush

Venus: When I was in middle school and high school, I didn't think a lot about boys and dating. I was very focused on school and tennis. But that Serena—now, she's another story! Ever since she was in the fourth grade, she's always had crushes on one guy or the other. But she didn't have any boyfriends. We weren't allowed to date until we were older. In that sense, we were kind of late bloomers.

Instead of focusing on love during my teenage years, I decided that my job was to learn as much as I could and do well in school so I'd be prepared for adulthood. I took the time to learn about myself—to figure out what I like and dislike, the things I'm good at, stuff I need to do better, the kinds of people I want to be around. Romance would distract from that so it would have to wait until later.

A teenage Venus and Serena take time to check out the sights in Melbourne, Australia.

"Since I didn't date boys, I learned to make dates with myself."

Since I didn't date boys, I learned to make dates with myself. And I still do! I schedule times when I explore things I've been curious about. As I travel I may go to an art museum I always wanted to visit or to study the fashions of the region. Sometimes I go alone, other times I go with friends or maybe someone from my family. This is another area where your parents or Dream Team can help: keeping their eyes open for neat things to do, getting tickets, driving and chaperoning, for instance.

Now that I'm an adult, having romantic relationships has become more important. I'm starting to develop crushes on guys. Crushes are *so much fun!* I love when someone who's handsome and nice smiles at me and has pretty eyes. And I like when someone thinks I'm cute and flirts a little bit. But ever since I started noticing guys, I've needed to make sure my romantic energy didn't get out of hand. I need to handle my chores and daily responsibilities whether or not someone is in my life.

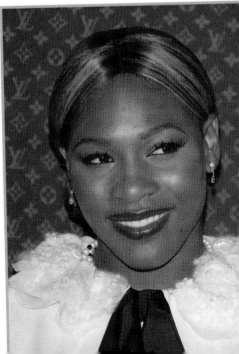

Serena at the Louis Vuitton United Cancer Front Gala, 2004.

serena: **When Venus,** my other sisters, and I were growing up, we didn't argue with our parents about not being able to date. That's just the way it was. We accepted it. Our parents had our best interests at heart, and we knew it. I didn't have my first boyfriend until I was eighteen years old. Until then, I always had guy friends just like I had girlfriends—buddies, partners,

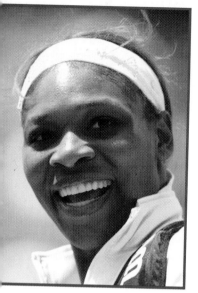

Serena smiles after a win at the 2004 French Open.

"Having friendships with people of both genders gives me a more complete outlook on everything."

pals, *amigos*, and chums. I think it was good for me then, and it still is now. I get to talk about and do different things when I'm with guys than when I'm with my girls. I really like getting to hear opinions from a male point of view. Fifty percent of the world is composed of people of the opposite sex. If I don't know what kinds of things are on their minds, I'll be missing out on half of life. Having friendships with people of both genders gives me a more complete outlook on everything.

I look for the same qualities in a guy as I do in girls. He has to be genuine and have a good heart and high morals. And it doesn't hurt if he has a good sense of humor, because I like to laugh a lot—all the time, if possible. I sometimes wish some of the people I knew had had the same family rule about age limits on dating that we did. They had some good times, but there was just so much pain involved in dating— who said what to whom, who cheated on whom, who went to what base, and who got pregnant. There were a lot of tears, arguments, dustups, and people coming to blows. Most of the time it seemed like someone's feelings were getting hurt.

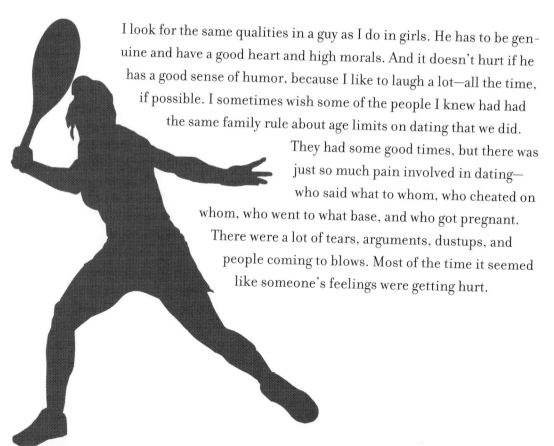

"Because we didn't have boyfriends, we were able to focus a lot more of our energy on ourselves."

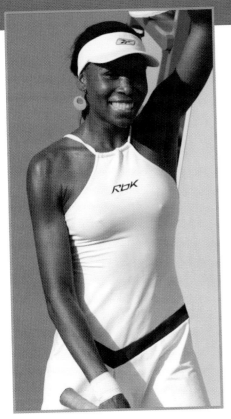

Venus acknowledges the crowd after a 2004 match in Dubai.

Meanwhile, back at the Williams household, Venus and I were feeling peaceful and focusing on achieving the dreams we had for our lives. Now, don't get me wrong. I'm not trying to say that the reason we became stars is because we didn't have boyfriends. But we *were* able to focus a lot more of our energy on ourselves. The areas that you focus your attention on are where you get results in life. I'm not sure where we would be if we had spent our teenage years ga-ga over cute guys. But I feel that we've gotten further in life because we waited until much later.

I'm sure this is what our parents had in mind when they set the "no dating" rule. Even though it restricted us at the time, I know they believe in falling in love. We wouldn't be here if they didn't already know a lot about the birds and the bees!

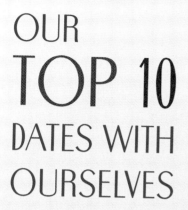

OUR
TOP 10
DATES WITH
OURSELVES

Forget about the mall and the pizza shop. The world has so much to offer, so step off the beaten path. Here are some great places to take yourself out on a date!

- an art, science, or natural history museum

- a museum that teaches you about your own ethnicity or culture

- a concert of any kind—R&B, rock, pop, hip-hop, opera, classical, jazz, blues, folk, or international music

- a nature center

- a walk or hike through a park

- a seat next to a lake or a river with your notebook, sketchbook, or journal

- a theater that plays documentary movies and films made in other countries and in different languages

- a local college so you can walk around and get familiar with what it feels like to be on a campus

- the local library or a bookstore

- a work environment that excites you. Intern-for-a-day at your dream job!

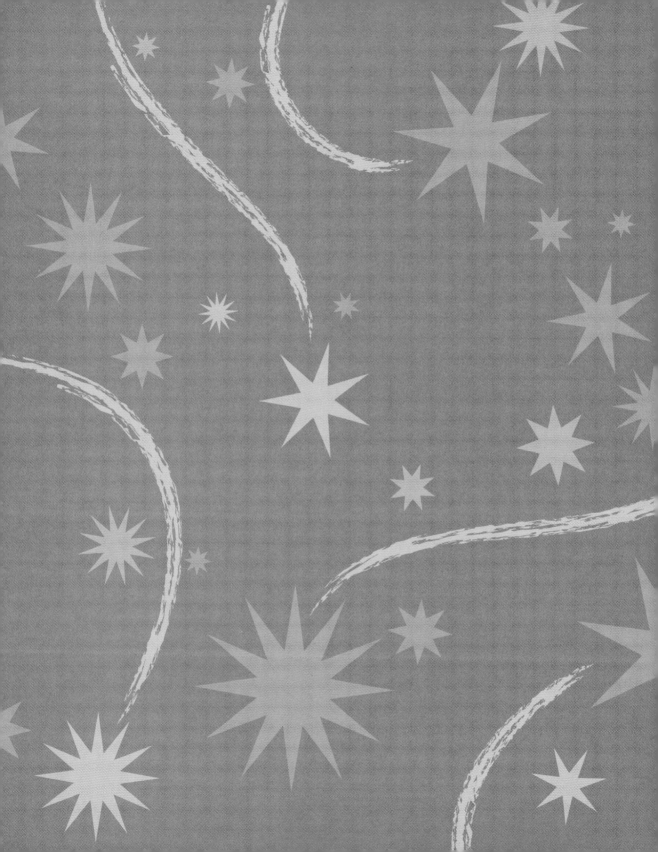

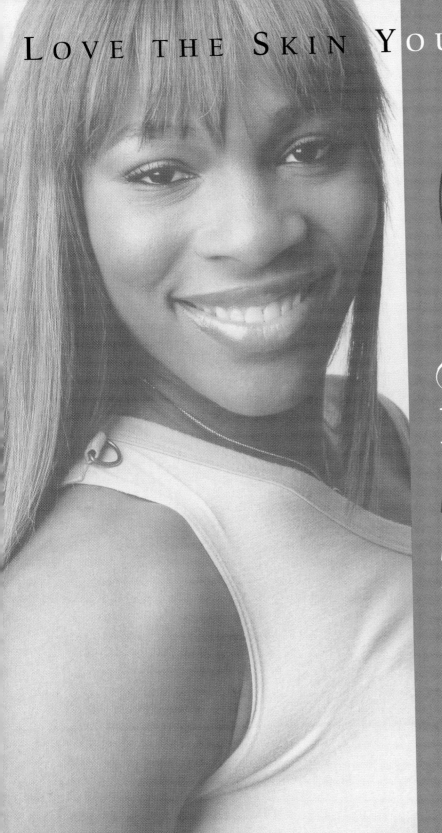

LOVE THE SKIN YOU'RE IN

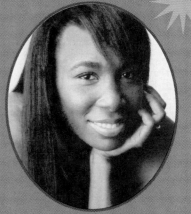

Sister Rule #7

MIRROR,
MIRROR, ON
THE WALL,
BEAUTY LIVES
INSIDE US ALL.

SERENA

love the skin you're in

Serena: When I became a teenager,
I experienced times when I felt insecure about my looks. I wished that my face were more attractive. At one point I thought I was a little pudgy and wished that I were slimmer. Later, I believed that my legs were too big and my body was too muscular.

During those years there were many times I wished that I could mix and match body parts with someone else. I would have given anything to have Venus's long and slender legs, my sister Lyndrea's tiny waist, my sister Isha's skin, and my sister Yetunde's eyes. Of course, that wasn't possible. Over time my physical features all caught up with one another and everything balanced out. As that happened, I started to come into my own and grow comfortable in my skin. At some point it just dawned on me that this is the body God gave me and I love and appreciate it no matter what. And who am I to complain? Not everyone has a healthy body or one that is fit and strong. These days, I'm grateful that I'm healthy. And I've accepted having a figure that is more curvy and muscular than long and slender and lean. These days, I'm very happy with who I am. I don't long to look like anyone but Serena.

My issues with body image are pretty common. At some point during their lives many of my friends—especially females—have felt uncomfortable about some aspect of their appearance. It's really hard not to have these feelings in this culture. We watch movies, videos, and commercials and read magazines

"This is the body God gave me and I love and appreciate it no matter what."

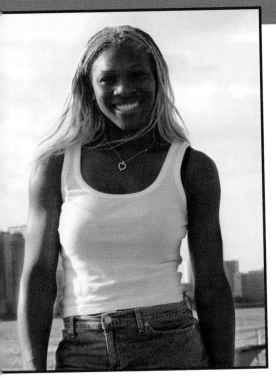

Serena at the beach.

that communicate a standard of beauty that hardly anyone can reach. Since I've appeared in a number of magazines—*Vibe, Vogue, Essence, Elle,* and *Sports Illustrated* to name a few—I can tell you that a lot more happens at photo shoots than is apparent when you're looking at the pictures. First, there's a whole crew of people whose sole job is to make you look beautiful. No matter what you look like when you show up—you can be a zit face who's gotten no sleep, and your hair can be all over your head—you're going to look like a million bucks because they spend several hours working on you. There's always at least one makeup artist to do your makeup perfectly, and a hairstylist who creates a hairstyle that enhances your face and the clothing you're modeling. They bring all their tools—makeup, brushes, curling irons, hair pieces, enough hair spray to make my dog look like a porcupine— every product you could ever imagine.

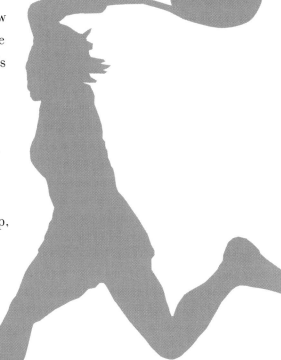

"At first, the tennis world didn't know what to make of our look."

After they're finished and the photographer is taking your picture, they hover around you like bumblebees. If even one hair moves out of place, they stop all the action and put it back. Wouldn't you look amazing all the time if you had a team of people following your every move, brushing new makeup on you if you start to sweat?

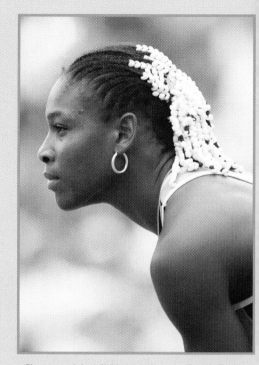

Playing with braided hair in the 1999 French Open.

And after all of that, when the pictures are developed a designer digitally alters them to get rid of dark circles and bags under eyes, make teeth appear whiter, and hide zits, moles, scars, and marks everyone has from falling off a bike when they were a kid. Because so many people are fooled into believing these images are real, a lot of people strive to obtain a look that's not achievable—well, unless you want to have a team of makeup artists following you around everywhere.

"We do everything we can to take care of ourselves."

Even then, you may look good on the outside but have a nasty personality. Real beauty comes from the inside out. So instead of feeling bad because we don't look like this silly standard or adopting unhealthy habits to try to make ourselves into something we're not, Venus and I do our best to be kind to the people we meet and work with the bodies God gave us. That means we do everything we can to take care of ourselves, and we find clothes that are flattering to our body types.

Venus and I have a lot of fun with fashion on the tennis court. When we started playing professionally we wore our hair braided with lots and lots of white beads in them. At first, the tennis world didn't know what to make of our look. Then, just when they had gotten used to it, we switched up and sported new styles. We have adopted different hairstyles ever since. We also try different fashions on the court. In the past, tennis players usually wore a lot of white and conservative styles and colors. We bring our flair to the sport by wearing new and exciting shapes, designs and colors that we think flatter our looks. Just because everyone else wears certain brands and styles of clothes doesn't mean that you have to follow their lead.

venus: **When Serena and I were** growing

up, our mom and dad didn't let us eat a lot of junk food— cookies, cakes, pies, presweetened cereals, candy, potato chips, pork rinds, and ice cream. In fact, they wouldn't

"When you're young you're training yourself to build healthy habits that you can follow for the rest of your life."

even bring it into the house. But as soon as I was old enough to get an allowance, I'd buy doughnuts from the ice cream truck. That wasn't the same as having access to junk food morning, noon, and night, but I still developed a taste for sweets. We were really lucky that our parents made us eat healthily. A balanced diet—fruits and vegetables, cereals and grains, dairy products and proteins—gave us lots of energy and made our bodies grow strong and healthy. Since we learned to eat right when we were younger, now that we're out on our own, we don't have too many bad eating habits to unlearn. We're very conscious of what we put into our mouths, even though we can eat anything we want. To have strong bodies and enough energy to play well—not to mention keep up with our busy schedules—we eat balanced meals that contain a lot of vitamins and minerals. Sorry to break the bad news to you: sugary foods, like candy bars, and foods high in fat, like potato chips, French fries, and frozen dinners, just don't make the cut.

Even though I take healthy eating very seriously, I do give myself fun days when I make frozen waffles or pancakes and syrup for breakfast or treat myself to a cup of hot chocolate. Or maybe I'll stop by a fast food restaurant and get a cheeseburger and French fries, or I'll order a pizza. Since balance is important, I don't

> "Exercise has great benefits: a strong body, a good
> self-image, good balance, and lifelong healthy habits."

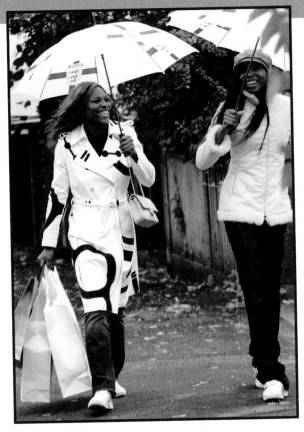

Venus and Serena on a shopping trip in London.

do this too often. These days I eat more healthily than ever. But back in the day, Serena and I were known to eat too many marshmallows and fruit roll-ups and to have an occasional chip binge. These kinds of foods tend to be high in fat and lower in vitamins and minerals than others. So if you eat too much of them you end up not taking good care of yourself. Remember, when you're young you're training yourself to build healthy habits that you can follow for the rest of your life.

I also try to practice the good habit of listening to my body and eating only when I'm hungry. That way, instead of living to eat, I eat to live. Otherwise, I'll just be eating to be eating, which means the food will be converted to fat because my body doesn't need the calories for fuel. Recently, I've been successful at breaking a bad eating habit. I used to live for sweets—doughnuts were the greatest! But sweets keep my body from performing at its peak. I realized that the longer I kept eating everything sugary in sight it would be

"When my body is strong, I also feel powerful in other areas of my life."

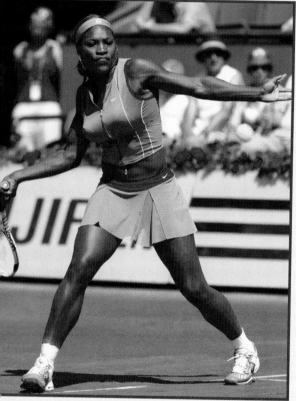

Serena prepares for a shot during the 2004 French Open.

harder and harder to break the habit. So I took the plunge and cut sugar out of my life. I didn't have anything unnaturally sweet for a long time. At first it was hard, but it got a lot easier. I did really well for a while. Instead of using sugar, I did things like sweeten my cereal with raisins and my lemonade with honey. But then I traveled to Australia and Japan and went totally out of control. I was in Australia for about a week, but while I was there I ate twelve pieces of apple pie. Then I went to Tokyo, where I pigged out on doughnuts! I just couldn't quit. I had a complete relapse into unhealthy eating habits. I knew I had to change. I had to regroup and try again. That happens some-times—you backslide into a bad habit. There's no sense in beating yourself up about it. Just pick a day and start over fresh!

serena: **On top of eating well,** it's important to stay active. If Venus and I ruled the world, everyone would participate in regular exercise. Exercise has great benefits: a strong body, a good self-image, good balance, and lifelong healthy habits. Working out also makes you feel confident in your body and your physical abilities. When I'm in my best shape, I can run forever on the tennis court. I don't have to worry about needing to cut the

"Health comes in all shapes and sizes. You don't have to look a certain way to be in shape."

point short so I can stop and catch my breath. I am able to challenge my opponent more. I feel as if I can run down any ball and within seconds be ready for the next thing to happen. When I'm fit I feel I can do *anything*. When I'm not in good enough shape, my legs get tired and my chest burns a lot. I go for ridiculous shots because I'm too exhausted to continue the point. Fortunately that hasn't happened often. And being in good shape has another reward: When my body is strong, I also feel powerful in other areas of my life.

But if you have this image of good health as tall and slim, you'd better look again. Health comes in all shapes and sizes. You don't have to look a certain way to be in shape. Fitness is personal. In our family we run the full spectrum of heights, weights, and bone structures. But even though we're built differently, our bodies are all beautiful. No matter our shape, what is important is that we're healthy. And to be healthy you have to be involved in some level of physical activity, which we all are.

Not everyone thinks being active is fun—which I can understand. While Venus and I both love to play tennis, we hate medicine balls and Thera-Bands and the kind of training we have to do off the court. We'd both rather sit on our tushes. But even when we have to run wind sprints in the sand or

"Being active is so fun . . . enjoy it!"

do other grueling workouts, after it's over we feel better. It's like, "Yeah, I'm bad now. I really got it done!" There are many different reasons why people don't work out. But being active is so fun, we want to encourage you to find ways to enjoy it!

venus: There is so much stuff you can do if you get out there and get moving. You may think that Serena and I have only played tennis. But back in the day I ran track, and we tried ballet, martial arts, riding bikes, yoga, double-dutch, cheerleading, and a whole bunch of other activities. Remember the song "Are You That Somebody?" by Aaliyah on the Dr. Doolittle soundtrack? We used to love it. We'd watch the video and try to do the dance. Or Michael Jackson's "Smooth Criminal"? We would imitate him and try to lean way over like he does in the video. But we couldn't do it without falling down, so we would take belts and ties and tilt each other over. In retrospect, it probably wasn't the safest thing, but it *is* what we used to do. These kinds of activities help keep you fit.

"You don't have to be great at the sport, just willing to have a great time!"

When we were teenagers, Serena and I also loved going surfing—just *loved* it! Since we were just learning, we wiped out a lot—trying to balance on a surfboard is really hard even when you're already athletic! I was always skinning an elbow or knee. But each of my scrapes came with a great story about my amazing surfing adventures! Here's one—but first the disclaimer "Don't Try This at Home." When I was about sixteen, a friend took Serena and me surfing along the Pacific Coast Highway outside Los Angeles. We were good swimmers so we figured we'd try it even though the shoreline was rocky. I thought I was getting in the ocean at the right time—between groups of waves, when I should have had time to paddle out to the place where the water was calm so I could catch an inbound swell. But I counted wrong and a set of waves came in while I was still heading out. They swept me back to the shore and banged me up against the rocks. Every time I tried to swim past them, they kept pushing me back into the cliff. Then it occurred to me that I didn't need to hold on to my board with my hands since it was attached to my leg with an ankle strap. With my hands and arms free I was able to swim as hard as I could past the waves, then I headed back to the beach so I could rest and laugh about my experience. Sure enough, when I got out of the water I had scraped my leg on the rocks! I was too tired to go back in, but I had gotten an excellent workout—and an important lesson

"If you put in the time and effort, you'll be rewarded with confidence and new physical abilities."

about the power of nature! Your exercise regimen doesn't have to be this adventurous; the point is to try something new and exciting and to have as much fun as you can. You don't have to be great at the sport, just willing to have a great time!

If you don't work out because you don't want to mess up or sweat out your hair, try out another style that makes working out easy. Why do you think Serena and I wear so many braided styles? Of course, we think they're cute, but also they make taking care of our hair and working out a whole lot easier. And here's a fitness tip that will help you stay fashionable: Make the day you do your cardiovascular activities (exercises that make you breathe hard and your heart pound) a day that you wash your hair.

serena: If you put in the time and effort, you'll be rewarded with confidence and new physical abilities. Even a little bit of effort in all of these areas—finding your own style, eating right, and becoming more physically fit—will help you develop strong self-esteem and a positive body image.

CAFÉ VENUS

*O*ut with the chips and candy bars! These foods I enjoy will give you energy to burn, whether on a regular day or one when you need to perform your best.

Regular Day

BREAKFAST:

◆ 1 piece of fruit OR 1 glass of orange juice (preferably fresh squeezed from the tree in our backyard) diluted with water to cut the sugar

   AND

◆ 1 bowl whole-grain cereal OR 1 bowl plain yogurt with fresh fruit, honey, and granola,

   AND

◆ Lots of water

LUNCH:

◆ 1 turkey sandwich on whole-grain bread with lettuce, tomato, and mustard

   OR

◆ 1 large salad containing lettuce, walnuts, raisins, feta cheese, olive oil, and lemon juice (grapes, sunflower seeds, and tuna fish are also fun ingredients)

   OR

◆ 1 piece grilled or broiled fish or barbecued chicken with fresh veggies like broccoli and a potato

DINNER:

◆ Same foods as lunch, plus brown rice

SNACK:

◆ Nuts and fruit (I love prunes and cherries)

   AND

◆ At least 2 liters of water drunk all day long

Game Day

Same foods as a regular day, although I may add some whole-wheat pasta with meat, marinara, or cream sauce, and a banana after my match and plenty of water

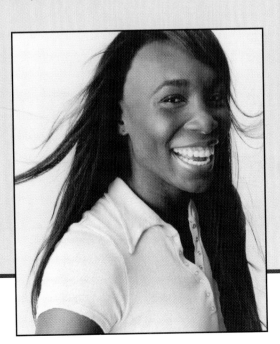

GET
MOVIN'!

Are you new to exercising or looking to improve your workout? If so, these tips will put you in high gear.

◆ **Make time.** Exercising is a habit we want you to adopt for life. Carve out at least thirty minutes four or more times a week.

◆ **Mix it up.** Alternate between activities like aerobics, baseball, basketball, biking, boxing, cheerleading, dancing, double-dutch, football, gymnastics, jogging, Pilates, skateboarding, skiing, snow-boarding, soccer, softball, surfing, swimming, tennis, track, volleyball, walking, weightlifting, and yoga.

◆ **Chill out.** Start slowly. Don't try to go hardcore and get fit in a day. You'll just end up disappointed in your-self. Take your time and build your strength and endurance gradually.

◆ **Maximize your workout.** Start by stretching your entire body—neck, arms and shoulders, torso, and legs. Strengthen your heart and lungs by doing activities, like running, playing soccer, or boxing, that cause your heart to beat harder. This can include walking as long as you move quickly enough that you have difficulty talking. And don't forget to lift weights. Strength training is especially important if you're trying to lose weight, since it causes your body to burn more calories, even when you're sleeping.

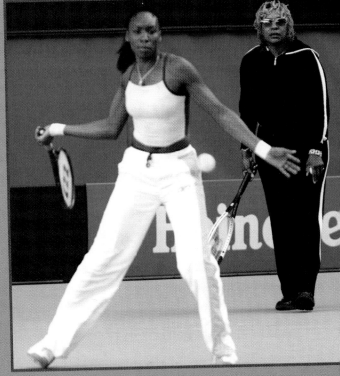

Oracene Price watches Venus practice her strokes before the 2003 Australian Open.

◆ **Get wet.** Sweat is your body's way of regulating its temperature. It cleans out your pores and removes toxins from your body. It's all good.

◆ **Expect soreness.** Your muscles will feel sore for several weeks after you start. This is healthy. They're getting used to moving. If sore muscles make you uncomfortable, take a relaxing bath with a cup or two of Epsom salts, available at the grocery store.

◆ **Up your game.** Set goals for yourself that push you beyond where you are now. If you can do only ten sit-ups a day this week, shoot for fifteen next week.

HYGIENE 101:
SO FRESH AND SO CLEAN

*N*othing will make other kids tease and not want to be around you faster than overlooking your personal hygiene. Don't make life hard on yourself. These basic grooming tips will keep you smelling and looking wonderful.

◆ **Bathing.** We bathe or take a shower every day. Because we live in Florida, where it can get very hot and humid, most days we shower twice. We also bathe more often if we've been involved in physical activity of any kind. Don't have showers at your school? Keep some deodorant (we call it anti-funk) in your locker at all times. It's also smart to keep a washcloth or wipes in your locker (a paper towel also works). You can wash your underarms and apply fresh deodorant. If you get sweaty between your legs, just do a wipe-down in a stall. Wipe everywhere—and we do mean everywhere! Don't forget one single spot. If you sweat a lot, keep an extra shirt in your locker. Take it from us: Having B.O. is the best way to get a bad rep!

◆ **Brushing and flossing.** We brush our teeth at least twice a day—morning and night. And flossing is a must. We don't want to end up with dragon breath. Wear braces, like Serena did? If so, brush more often. Bottom line: Brush and floss every tooth you want to keep.

◆ **Female cleanliness.** A lot of you are at the age where you're starting to have your period. If so, always change your pad or tampon at least every three to four hours.

◆ **Hair care.** It's important to wash your hair at least once or twice a week. If you sweat a lot or work out, you may want to wash it more often. User-friendly hairstyles like short cuts and braids can make life a lot easier. And condition, condition, condition. Make "hair conditioner" your middle name.

◆ **Skin care.** We wash our faces at least twice a day—when we wake up and at bedtime. We wash gently, so we don't stretch our skin. Got zits? We have them, too, from time to time. But we don't pop them because we don't want to get marks and scars. See a dermatologist if they become a nuisance. Don't stress; they will clear up. And whenever you go outside, apply sunscreen with an SPF of at least 15. The ozone layer is thinning, so you need protection whether your skin color is ivory or ebony.

◆ **Undergarments.** Wear clean underwear every day! This is a must—even if that means you have to wash your clothes out in the sink at night. You can use a light detergent or soap. It's okay to repeat your bra, but be sure to wash it at least once a week.

◆ **Washing your clothes.** Is your dirty-clothes hamper overflowing? Now that you're getting older, don't rely on your parents to keep up with your laundry. Start washing your own clothes, and they will be ready when you need them. As long as they smell fresh and look clean, we repeat our clothes without washing them every time.

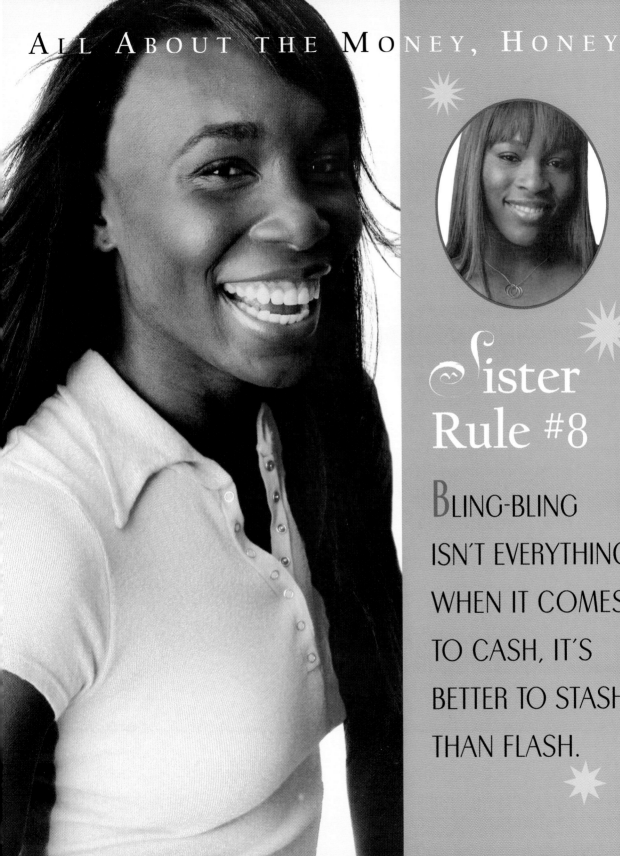

ALL ABOUT THE MONEY, HONEY

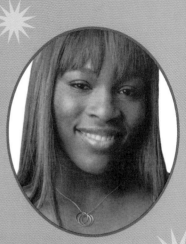

Sister Rule #8

BLING-BLING ISN'T EVERYTHING. WHEN IT COMES TO CASH, IT'S BETTER TO STASH THAN FLASH.

VENUS

all about the money, honey

*V*enus: **When I was ten years old** and Serena was eight or nine, our parents started giving us an allowance of five dollars a week. Serena spent almost all of her money buying lunch at school and snacks. Since lunch cost only forty cents a day, she was blowing three dollars a week on the ice cream truck. She was often broke by Wednesday. Every now and then I would have to help her out. One time I stumbled across her looking pitiful in the lunch line. When she told me she was broke and that the only thing available as a free lunch was a peanut butter and jelly sandwich, I gave her *my* lunch money and ate the peanut butter sandwich myself.

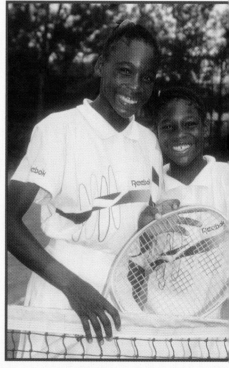

Young sisters on the court in Florida

Even though I rescued her from her poor money management many times back in the day, I wasn't much better at it than she was. I would spend most of my allowance on doughnuts—which I *loved*— and grab bags I bought from the ice cream truck.

"Every morning while Venus and I slept, Lyn got up and went to work."

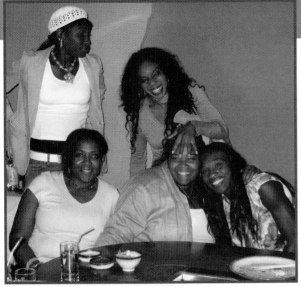

The Williams sisters together in Wimbledon, 2003.

Those grab bags were one big waste of money when they were full of things I didn't like. And even when I got good treats, they were gone in a matter of minutes.

serena: While

Venus and I were scroung-ing around broke, our sister Lyndrea, who's two years older than Venus, was handling her business. Lyn still bought lunches at school and treated herself to goodies from time to time, but she put herself on a budget. Venus and I didn't notice this until the day Lyn walked in the house wearing a great new pair of shoes. We were stunned. We couldn't figure out how she had got-ten them. Then Lyn explained that she had been saving every spare penny she had. After a while the money added up and she was able to indulge herself with a more long-lasting possession.

A few years later Lyn taught us another important lesson about money. When we were teenagers, she found a summer job. Every morning while Venus and I slept, Lyn got up and went to work. We just didn't get what the big deal was about work—that is, until she came home with shopping bags full of great outfits for school. That's when it

"Lyn and Yetunde taught us a lot about hard work, saving, and spending."

finally made sense to us: Money is a tool that can help you improve your life and become more independent—but you have to work hard and make sacrifices to earn it.

Lyn had learned to be industrious from our mom, who worked long hours as a nurse, and our oldest sister, Yetunde. Yetunde was smart about saving her money and loved being able to afford some things for herself while also being generous with us. Sometimes we would hear her telling one of her friends, "No, I can't go out tonight. I have to save my money. I want to buy some clothes for my sisters."

It may have taken a little while for the learning to sink in, but our experiences with Lyn and Yetunde taught us a lot about hard work, saving, and spending. Spending our money on snacks at school and ice cream grab bags was fun, but the things we bought and the thrills that came with them didn't last very long. By being industrious, saving, and practicing self-control, you can purchase things that are more meaningful to you, last longer, and improve your life, just as Lyndrea did.

venus: Serena and I learned these principles from Yetunde, Lyndrea, and other members of our Dream Team and diligently applied them to our lives. Today our years of working hard and making sacrifices so that we could become tennis cham-

"Today our years of working hard and making sacrifices . . . have paid off for us in more ways than we ever imagined."

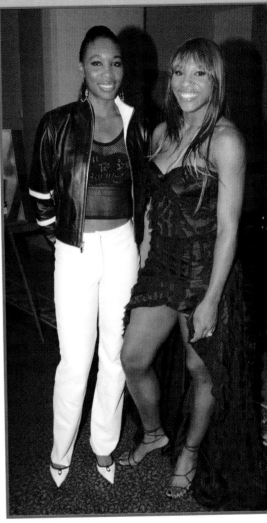

Venus and Serena at a Women's Tennis Association fashion show.

pions have paid off for us in more ways than we ever imagined. Our success has made us millionaires. Serena and I share a wonderful house and have other nice possessions. We're able to pay for our own college educations; hire the coaches, agents, and trainers we need to keep us physically and financially fit; plus pay expenses like airplane tickets and hotel bills as we pursue our careers.

You may be familiar with the very visible part of our lives—the "flash"—the tennis tournaments, endorsement deals, and award shows and fundraisers we go to from time to time. But the flash isn't everything or even the most important part of our lives. The work we do behind the scenes isn't very sexy or exciting, but it helps us prosper personally and professionally. These areas of our lives are like our own private "stash" because they're socked away from public view but always working for us.

People see Serena and me attending events like the MTV music awards and think that every day in our lives is as exciting and glamorous as that. *We wish!* She and I love those events because they are so exciting! But we spend most of our days working and educating ourselves. Our work includes practicing

"We're preparing ourselves today for our lives in the future."

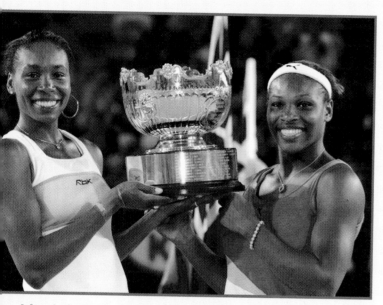

Lifting the doubles trophy at the 2003 Australian Open.

tennis, training and conditioning our bodies, managing our second jobs, studying, and getting enough rest. We work very, very hard, day in and day out. As athletes we have a limited number of years that our bodies are in their prime and healthy. Eventually the next generation of women will rise to the top of the tennis world or we'll get injured or decide to retire. That's how life is when you play pro sports or are an actor or entertainer— there's no guarantee that any of us will make a lot of money forever.

Serena and I work as much as we can while our names are hot. Even though we have fabulous lives, we don't live flashy lifestyles. Instead, we stay focused on our stash—our education, managing our money, and following through on our plans. We take advantage of our earning power both on and off the court by winning as many tournaments as we can and getting product endorsement deals. Serena and I also hold down second and third jobs—acting, designing clothes, and running Aneres and V Starr Interiors. We do all this because we love it, and because we're preparing ourselves today for our lives in the future.

"Very few people get super-rich."

We also watch what we spend. We don't blow our money wastefully or live above our heads. I am a nickel-and-dimer. Contrary to what you may think, I don't own many designer clothes. I've been known to purchase a well-made T-shirt from the drugstore for ten dollars and wear it to death. Serena lives on a budget and has her business manager give her an allowance. Rather than wasting our money on "bling-bling" and other frivolous things, we save, buy stocks and bonds, purchase real estate, and make other investments that will help us earn money long after our tennis years are over. There's nothing more embarrassing for a celebrity than to have a lot of money, spend it foolishly, and end up with nothing.

We've also made many sacrifices to build the lives we have today. Somebody asked me recently whether I ever think about getting married. I told them that I'm already married—to tennis. Serena and I can't make any decisions in our personal lives without considering how they will impact our work schedules—which are sometimes just grinding. In our world there's no such thing as saying "I'm tired." We might have enough *money* to take vacations or to spend the week at a spa, but in actuality we have very little *time* for relaxation. Now, don't get me wrong, I'm not complaining. We love playing tennis and the life that comes with being champs. But since the "lifestyles of the rich and famous" are

"Rather than wasting our money on 'bling-bling' and other frivolous things, we save."

idealized on TV and so many people aspire to be superstars, we want to be honest about what it means for us. There is more than one side of the "glamorous life" that athletes and entertainers live. The public doesn't always get to see the incredible hours and strenuous work that take place behind the scenes.

serena: Because television promotes the far-out aspects of some celebrities' lifestyles, it's easy to mistakenly believe that it's important to have lots of cash, cribs, cars, clothes, and ice. Having money *is* essential. You need it to do important things like eat, and pay rent and utility bills. And it gives you more

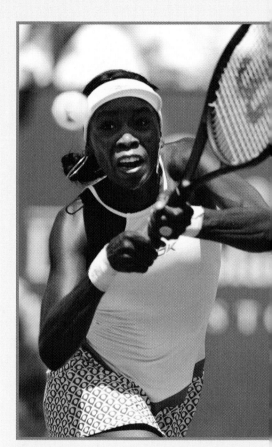

Venus tracking the ball at the 2004 Family Circle Cup semifinal in South Carolina.

options in life, like the chance to go to better schools, travel, or go to college. But getting rich is not one of the most important things you need to accomplish in life—it's not even close! No matter what hype you see on TV, very few people get super-rich. So, since

"Getting rich is not one of the most important things you need to accomplish in life—it's not even close!"

money doesn't grow on trees, it's important to be financially responsible. You can create a fun and exciting future whether or not you're loaded. Of course, you have to work hard and squirrel away your funds instead of spending them all at the mall. But when you save some money every week from your allowance, babysitting, or job, you're preparing for your life and you can really feel proud of that. By stashing your funds for things that are meaningful—like music lessons or an instrument, basketball camp, or a trip to France with your French class—you can learn things and have experiences that will stay with you forever. These types of expenses are "investments"—the type of spending that builds you up and benefits you for a long period of time.

One of the best investments you can make is to start early saving money for college. Ask your parents if they will help you open a bank account. Then set a goal to put a certain amount of money in it every month—even five or ten dollars. You'll have the satisfaction of seeing your money grow—both the cash you save and the money you earn as the bank pays you interest. You'll receive a bank statement in the mail every month that you'll get to learn how to read. And you'll feel satisfied knowing that you're taking care of business by setting aside funds for an exciting future.

"One of the best investments you can make is to start early saving money for college."

But we know that not everyone has enough money to open a savings account. If you don't, it's really important that you do a good job of managing the educational part of your stash. Getting a good education paves the way to higher-paying jobs and a college degree. So whatever you do, don't overlook your books. Try to get the highest grades you can—all A's and B's if possible. And make sure to ask one of your school counselors to be on your Dream Team. You'll need them to help you plan to take the right classes and apply for college.

Even though you might think that becoming rich can solve all your problems, it can't. Venus and I know that no amount of our cash can buy the most important things in life: love, family, friendship, good health, and happiness. And it can't purchase the satisfaction you feel when you've worked hard, achieved your goals, and become the best at something.

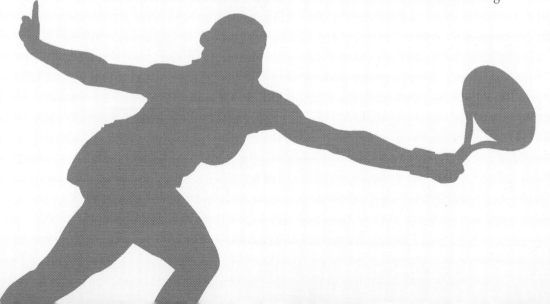

✳ TRY MY SNEAKERS ON FOR SIZE ✳

Venus: I know what you see on television, but most of my life isn't as elegant as you may think. There is no cute mascot to cheer "Go, Venus! You are the greatest player in the history of the world!" while I hit thousands of practice balls each day in the sweltering Florida heat and humidity. No fans are there to cheer me on when I have to run so many wind sprints that I feel like I'm going to drop. No one is spritzing me with cool water or fanning me with palm leaves or feeding me grapes when I take breaks during practice. Most days, Serena and I are our own fan club as we go to work, practice our game, and push ourselves to higher levels. Here's how I spend a typical day when I'm not in the public eye.

- **7:00 a.m.** Wake up, shower, eat, and hop on the Internet to research whatever I'm studying at the moment. If I have a lot of studying to do, sometimes I'll get up earlier.

- **8:00 a.m.** Practice tennis (4 hours)

- **12:00 noon** Eat lunch (1 hour)

- **1:00 p.m.** Perform strength-training and conditioning exercises (2 hours)

- **3:00 p.m.** Perform stretching exercises and ice down the sore parts of my body (1 hour)

- **4:00 p.m.** Work at the offices of V Starr Interiors (2 or 3 hours)

- **7:00 p.m.** Eat dinner and go home to prepare for the next day

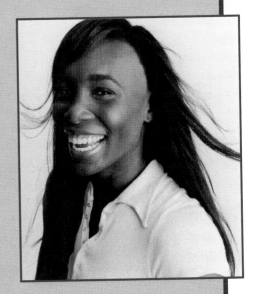

VIDEOS
AREN'T REAL

*S*erena: **If you're like many people,**
music videos (and celebrity "reality" TV shows) may have
made you believe that the lifestyles and extravagant activities they depict are common in real life. When you're rich
you *do* get to do and see some pretty incredible things,
and, yes, some of them are shown in videos. But I don't
know any successful athlete or entertainer who spends life
draped in diamonds and lounging in hot tubs surrounded
by half-naked women or men. I *do* know what happens on
a video shoot, though, since I made a cameo appearance in
one before, along with several other female athletes.

**Videos—just like photos in magazines—don't represent
real life.** Most of the things you see in them cannot be
attained. That's because videos are actually a fantasy product, just like Cinderella or another fairy tale, that a large
team of people came together to make. Behind the scenes
there are a whole lot of people whose jobs are to create an
illusion: makeup artists, set designers, clothing stylists,
hair stylists, florists, jewelers, prop artists, sponsors, and
companies that want their products seen, for example.
And that's all before the singers, musicians, dancers, and
other people who are actually *in* the video even show up.

Videos last for only a few minutes, but they may take days to film and sometimes months to produce. The dancers and extras who are in them may have to endure long hours for little pay. The stars work hard, too, but they're taken care of very well. They spend hours in hair and makeup so they can look as good as they do, and a stylist has spent days searching for the perfect clothes and jewelry for them to wear. Afterwards designers touch up the image digitally so the artist looks just right. If a team of people focused that hard on you, you'd look amazing, too!

You know that really cool set they've constructed? Well, after the video ends it comes down, and all the props that were rented for the shoot—the expensive furniture, the Escalades, the private jets—go back to wherever they came from. Everyone takes off their makeup, wigs, and designer clothing. The stylist who got the gear and shoes packs them up and takes them back to the showroom. The half-naked people who've been cavorting around put on their T-shirts and jeans and go back to their day jobs. The people who own the awesome crib where the video was shot get their house and hot tub back. And representatives for the jeweler walk right up to you, take their diamonds off you, and return them to the store.

Just as videos are flash, so are many of the glamorous aspects of Venus's and my lives. Next time you see us all decked out at an awards show, know that we get to be princesses for only a night. Then we go back home and get some sleep so we're ready for practice in the morning.

STEP BACK, SETBACKS!

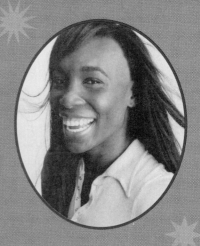

Sister Rule #9

CHALLENGES?
BRING 'EM ON!
I KEEP MY EYES
ON THE BALL
AND MY HEAD
IN THE GAME
OF LIFE.

SERENA

Serena: If there's something Venus and I know how to do really well, it's come back from behind. Both of us have been in some really thrilling matches where we dug ourselves into a hole by letting our opponent get ahead of us but climbed out and were able to win. In 2000, Venus was off the tour for six months, suffering with tendinitis. Experts in the tennis world were wondering if she'd be able to regain her form. But she returned and became better than ever. Venus won Wimbledon in both singles and in doubles (she and I were partners). She beat me in the finals of the U.S. Open. Then, she won two Olympic Gold Medals, and was chosen as *Sports Illustrated* magazine's Sportswoman of the Year.

Venus: Serena's had some pretty amazing comebacks herself. In the 2003 Australian Open, she played a fantastic semifinal match against a great player named Kim Clijsters, where she fended off two match points—that means that she was one point away from losing the match on two different occasions—and came from four games behind in the third set to win 4-6, 6-3, 7-5. Then she beat me to win the whole thing.

"The only thing that would help was to take time off from the tour to heal."

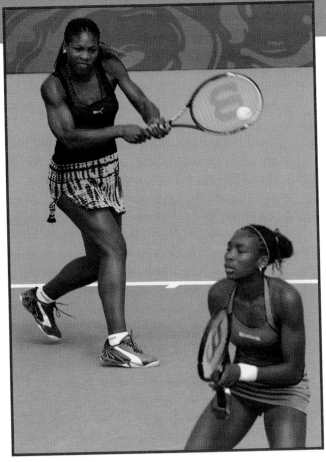

Playing doubles in the 2000 Olympics.

But in 2003 we both encountered challenges that we had never experienced before—really serious injuries. Until that point, we had been winning a lot and basically getting what we wanted professionally, so it was the first time we experienced major discouragement in our careers. That spring, I pulled one of my stomach muscles. I played several tournaments with my abs taped up for support. But when I lost to Serena in the finals at Wimbledon in the summer, they hurt so bad I could hardly stand up straight. I couldn't even pick up my gym bag. It was obvious that the only thing that would help was to take time off from the tour to heal. I was really disappointed. I had been playing well and came to Wimbledon believing I would win. Now I wouldn't go home with a Wimbledon trophy, *and* my tennis ranking would go down.

"I had worked hard to get to the top, and naturally I wanted to stay there."

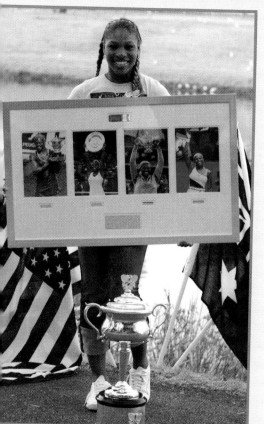

The Serena Slam.

serena: Around the time that Venus got hurt, I experienced major disappointment, too. I was at the peak of my career and ranked number one in the world. She and I had just made world history by being the first sisters to appear in the finals of four consecutive major tournaments: the 2002 French Open, Wimbledon, the U.S. Open, and the 2003 Australian Open. I won all four matches, creating the Serena Slam—what I call it when I win all four major tournaments in a row!—when a nagging injury in my knee started feeling uncomfortable. My doctors told me that I would have to have an operation. After the surgery I wouldn't be able to play tennis for months—I would only be able to do stretching and strengthening exercises. Needless to say, that wasn't what I wanted to hear. I had worked hard to get to the top, and naturally I wanted to stay there. Now, another player would take over my number one ranking. But I knew I had to take care of my body. I didn't want to continue to play and risk injuring myself worse.

As disappointed as I was, I remembered something very important our father had taught us to remember when things go wrong: No matter what you do and how hard you try, you can never turn back time—it's impossible! So I knew there was no use second-

"I . . . accept what has happened, quickly figure out what I need to do differently, make the change, and move on."

guessing my decision not to withdraw from any tournaments to rest my knee when I first got injured several months earlier.

I keep this thought—that you can't turn back time—in mind whenever things don't go my way in life or I get behind in a match. Instead of obsessing about things that are over, I focus on keeping my mind in the present moment so that I'm able to make good choices moving forward. It doesn't do any good to run an instant replay of any shot or situation over and over in my head. If I'm not paying attention now because I'm thinking about something in the past, I won't make the right choices for my future. The best thing I can do is accept what has happened, quickly figure out what I need to do differently, make the change, and move on.

venus: Sometimes life deals you

blows that can knock you to your knees. But no matter what happens, we all have to get up and move forward. Life goes on. That's why I think everyone needs a strategy to deal with difficulties. The first thing Serena and I do is turn to our spiritual roots. We don't have to turn very far, since we practice our religion faithfully. When I encounter problems in a specific area, I look for passages in

"Things are almost never as bad as we imagine them to be."

the Bible for guidance on dealing with that issue— scripture about endurance, strength, or courage.

The next thing I do is put the situation in perspective. Things are almost never as bad as we imagine them to be. I've experienced times when I was still all embarrassed about something and was creating all this drama in my head, but everyone else had moved on. Writing down your feelings in a notebook or journal can help clear out negative thoughts and emotions that keep you feeling stuck. If you don't have a lot of privacy, write down your thoughts and throw them away or tear the paper up and flush it down the toilet.

I also look for the bright side of the situation. No matter what frustrating, disappointing, or even bad thing has happened, I'm still going to be here and have to deal with it, so I might as well figure out how to turn my negative experience into a positive one. I decided to look at my stomach injury as a blessing that will lengthen my career. And rather than getting down in the dumps, I took advantage of the downtime to explore myself. There is so much stuff that I love to do but don't have enough time to enjoy when I'm touring—like working on my interior design business.

And it's really important to focus harder than ever on building yourself into who you want to be. When I wasn't able to play, I went to rehab to

"You can't let gossip and the negative opinions of other people pressure you into making decisions."

strengthen my body. Even though it's not as fun as playing tennis, rehab was a part of getting my body healthy and back in shape. I paid attention and applied myself. Between workouts I didn't sit around idle just because things weren't going my way. I took steps to stay motivated and excited by enjoying other areas of my life even through that rough stretch.

serena: Like Venus, while I was injured

I worked hard to help my knee heal and to get my body back in shape. Like her, I focused on other aspects of my career—I handled my endorsements, designed clothes, studied acting, got a part on a television show, and had fun. Because it took my knee longer to heal than people expected and I was involved in some very visible activities like fashion shows and acting, a lot of people speculated that I had lost interested in tennis. Others criticized how I was managing my career. And many people wondered out loud if I would ever regain my form and come back to dominate the game. Through all of this speculation and nay-saying, Serena stayed focused on Serena. As I told you before, you can't let gossip and the negative opinions of other people pressure you into making decisions or change how you live your life.

Finally, after eight months off the tennis tour, my knee had healed; I was back in shape and able to compete again. I had been practicing hard and was in great condition, so I was really, really excited about playing in tournaments again. My first—the

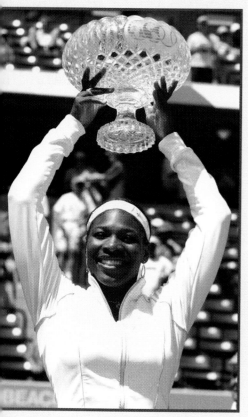

A happy Serena with the 2004 NASDAQ trophy.

"I couldn't believe I had won the first tournament I played in after coming back!"

NASDAQ 100—was held in Key Biscayne, Florida, pretty close to where I live. In my first match, I played pretty well, even though I was much more nervous than I usually am and my game was a little bit rusty from not playing in matches. The crowd was in my corner, which was great, and I was really relieved when I won. In my second match I played even better. I didn't make as many mistakes or feel anywhere near as nervous. Each day of the tournament my game improved and my nerves calmed down. My confidence grew. I even made it to the finals! I was really happy to get there, and was shocked that I won easily—6-1, 6-1—over a strong opponent. She didn't have her best day. Still, I couldn't believe I had won the first tournament I played in after coming back!

VENUS: My comeback didn't begin quite as easily as

Serena's did. About six months after I injured myself, my abs had healed and I was in fantastic shape. I played pretty well for someone who hadn't competed in six months, and I won an exhibition tournament in Hong Kong. But when I played in a tournament in Tokyo, I injured my knee. Then when I got to my next tournament—the Australian Open, one of the Grand Slam tournaments—I twisted my ankle *and* aggravated my knee. It really hurt, and it was hard to move around. Because of that, I got beat pretty early in the

"I decided that if I was to get out of this rut, I needed to go back to the beginning and focus on the basics."

tournament, which left me feeling shocked and disappointed. Australia is beautiful, but I went there to win the tournament, not to be a tourist.

My aches and pains kept nagging me during the beginning of the year. It would have been one thing to have one injury and get it over with. But to have all these injuries that were pretty debilitating and wouldn't go away— well, that was tough. And the more days I was injured and couldn't practice, the more I started getting out of shape. When I *was* able to play in tournaments, I wasn't up to par physically and didn't quite have the confidence I needed to hit my pressure shots. Of course, the more injuries I got and the more I struggled in matches, the more people in the tennis world started questioning whether I'd be able to come back. I shut them out and kept right on trying my hardest.

At the NASDAQ tournament, a few things finally started clicking. I made it to the quarterfinals, where I came from behind on a really good player and thought I would win. But I was still a little rusty from my long layoff and couldn't hold on to my lead under pressure. Serena won the tournament— and this time it wasn't because she beat me in the finals; it's because I didn't make it to the finals. I was mad at myself because I felt that I should have been there. That's when I had to dig even deeper within myself. I decided that if I was to get out of this rut, I needed to go back

"Superstars have to work hard and persevere through challenges just like everybody else does."

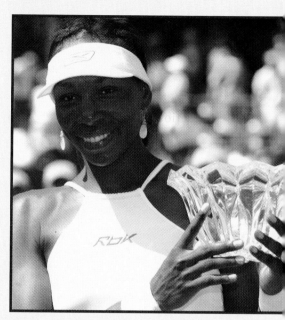

Venus prevails in the 2004 Family Circle Cup.

to the beginning and focus on the basics. So while everyone was out to dinner celebrating Serena's victory, Venus was back out on the tennis court practicing her strokes. It wasn't as fun as going out to eat, but it's what I had to do to get over the hump.

Fortunately, my diligence paid off. My injuries started to heal and my game began to come together. Before I knew it I had won two tournaments in a row, the Family Circle Cup in South Carolina and the J&S Cup in Poland—both on clay, my most difficult surface! In the third tournament, which took place in Germany, I made it to the semifinals, where I had a really tough match. I got behind 0-3 in the third set before I focused my mind and emotions and made a comeback. I won 6-4 in that last set and reached the finals! Unfortunately, during the last game of the match I hurt my ankle again. By the end of the day I was on crutches. I had to forfeit the finals without even playing. That's the worst—to give your opponent a victory without even making them play. Needless to say, I was very disappointed. But the ball doesn't always bounce your way.

"Stay focused on your dreams; keep your spirits high and your head in the game of life!"

Until this point, I'd been blessed not to have experienced this kind of discouragement in my career. I've had to keep working hard and not start crying and whining. When you feel like a victim and you have no control over the situation, that's when things really get bad. I focus on taking charge of the things that I have control over. Even though I have had bad moments and days, I always get myself back on track, fighting and working hard.

serena: **I wish that things had continued** to go easily during my comeback. Even though I won my first tournament after coming back, I experienced some disappointment, too. My knee started feeling sore again and my doctor advised me to slow down, that I was playing too much. I had to withdraw from two tournaments. In my next one, the Italian Open, I lost to Jennifer Capriati, one of my archrivals, in the semifinals. I always want to win, of course, but overall I'm happy with how I played her and she's a wonderful competitor.

Sometimes it's easy to come back from a loss or a mistake. Other times, coming back takes time. You have to hang in there, focus on the fundamentals and be patient with yourself. Superstars have to work hard and persevere through challenges just like everybody else does. The important thing is to stay focused on your dreams; keep your spirits high and your head in the game of life!

WHEN LIFE HANDS YOU LEMONS. . .

Venus: **Lemonade is one** of Serena's favorite drinks—which makes sense, since she sure does know how to make something sweet out of a sour situation. That's something that our parents always told us: when life hands you lemons, make lemonade. Back when we were teenagers, Serena and I were skateboarding together. I was always too scared to try a lot of new things, but that Serena . . . she was trying something kind of risky, when all of a sudden she wiped out. She tried to cushion her fall with her hands. But when she got up, her wrist was all banged up. This created a huge problem. In tennis your wrists need to be strong so you can hold the racquet firmly when you hit ground strokes and return serves that come at you at a hundred miles an hour. With her wrist hurt Serena could hardly hit her backhand—and she had a big tournament coming up in Zurich, Switzerland!

Rather than withdraw from the tournament, which would have made sense, Serena devised a strategy for dealing with her setback: Whenever her opponent would hit the ball to her backhand side, she would run around it and hit a forehand instead. Obviously, she couldn't do that with every shot—but she would try, she said. And she would pound it as hard as she could, so her opponent couldn't hit the ball back. When match day came, each time she hit a forehand—whether she ran around a backhand or the ball had been hit to her forehand side—she rocketed the ball back as hard as she could. And that's the inside scoop on how Serena Williams developed the killer forehand that terrorizes opponents from all over the world—by running around her backhand because she was too hurt to hit it. You heard it here first, folks!

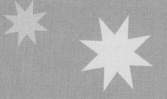

IT'S BETTER TO GIVE

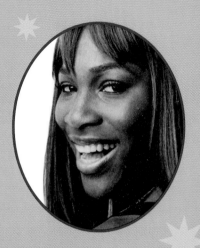

Sister Rule #10

YOU DON'T HAVE TO BE RICH OR FAMOUS TO SHARE YOUR BLESSINGS.

VENUS

it's better to give

𝒱enus: **When Serena was six years old** and I was seven or eight, my parents, all my sisters, and I went to a tennis clinic in Los Angeles hosted by Billie Jean King. Billie Jean is a famous tennis player who was once the best in the world. She grew up in Los Angeles and held the clinic there because she wanted to give back to the city that helped her become a superstar.

During the clinic, while we were practicing our shots, Billie Jean complimented my strokes. More than fifteen years have passed since that clinic, but I've never, ever forgotten her praise, and for some reason she remembers meeting me, too. The knowledge I got from her camp really helped my game. I was so inspired by the fact she had noticed me that I thought I could do anything. Ever since then I've always said, "When I grow up I'm going to do something like that for someone else."

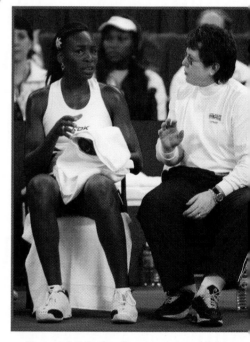

Venus with Billie Jean King during a 2003 Fed Cup match.

"We are all here to help one another."

serena: Two years later, when I was eight, Venus and I had the chance to meet Zena Garrison at a clinic our family drove to in Houston. Zena was a tennis champion, and I know she was really, really busy, but she still took the time to meet with us even though we weren't famous. I was just this little kid who, for some reason, thought I was good enough to beat her. I never forgot the experience or how nice she was to me—although when I hit with her, I quickly found out that I had absolutely no chance of winning!

venus: Serena and I had a great time at these clinics, which changed our lives forever. Being generous, like Billie Jean and Zena were with us, is an important part of being human. We are all here to help one another. And giving to others is another important way that we can learn about ourselves. The Bible teaches us that Jesus came so that he could help people, not so that people could help Him. I guess that's why it also tells us that it's better to give than to receive.

Serena and I share our blessings in life in some very basic ways. First, we show our gratitude to God by being generous in our spiritual community. Next, we look out for our Dream Team. We repay our parents for the love and sacrifices they've made for our family by making their lives a little easier. And since we couldn't have succeeded

"We get involved with lots of programs that help kids do better in school and go on to college."

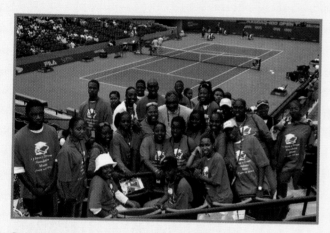

Richard Williams and students from the "I Have a Dream" Foundation at the 2004 NASDAQ tournament.

without our sisters' support—and since they also help us manage our personal and business affairs and sometimes accompany us on the road—we compensate them for their work and help them out from time to time. We don't think they need a handout, though. They have their own skills and talents and stand on their own two feet. We've also bought a home for our grandmother.

Remember the things we told you about getting a good education and going to college? We get involved with lots of programs that help kids do better in school and go on to college. In our neighborhood in Los Angeles where we grew up, we give back by going to our old schools and doing tennis clinics. We also support the Venus and Serena Williams Tutorial/Tennis Academy there. It helps inner-city high school tennis players improve their skills on the court and prepare to continue their schooling. We love helping these kids, especially since they remind us of ourselves when we were younger—outside of tennis inner circles, but hungry for success and highly motivated. They are determined to practice even though the tennis courts they play on are usually not in the best shape. Many of them have taught themselves to play, just like our father taught himself. Lots of times the high schools these kids go to don't even have tennis teams. Because of that they don't get the

> "We know that little gestures like these—that are so easy for us to make—can make all the difference in a young person's life."

coaching, experience playing in matches, or exposure that other kids get, and their games may not be quite as polished as kids who have coaches or can pay for lessons. They can't always afford to get a good tennis racquet and shoes or to pay to enter tournaments that will help them get ranked and noticed by college coaches. The odds are against them, yet they still keep trying.

These kids are perfect examples of people who stay focused on their dreams no matter what circumstances they encounter in life. That's why we lend them a hand by providing them with tennis coaching, resources to enter tournaments, tutoring, and other academic assistance, such as prep classes for college entrance exams and seminars on different careers. Sometimes we surprise the kids by showing up to practice or study with them. And we bring some of the kids to our matches when we're playing in L.A. We know that little gestures like these—that are so easy for us to make—can make all the difference in a young person's life.

We also invite kids to see us play when we're in Florida, where we live now. Remember Serena's comeback tournament where she won the NASDAQ 100 in Key Biscayne? Well, a few months earlier I had spoken to about a hundred young people

"I feel blessed that my life is an example to other people of how to achieve their dreams."

who are part of the "I Have a Dream" Foundation. The Foundation is really cool because it helps kids from low-income neighborhoods around the country—in this case, in Miami—by supporting them from kindergarten on with mentoring, tutoring, and other assistance, like funding to help them afford college. When Serena and I played in the NASDAQ, I invited some of the Dreamers, as they are called, to come and cheer us on. I've started developing relationships with a few of the kids, so when I see them, I can ask them about what's going on in their lives. It's great! One of the girls wants to study design, so she asks me a lot of questions about where she should go to school and how to get scholarship money. It feels wonderful to see her eyes light up when I tell her that she can do it. I feel blessed that my life is an example to other people of how to achieve their dreams. And it's exciting that I know enough about fashion that I can help someone else even though I'm at the beginning of my career and haven't finished my education. Everyone has something to offer someone else and it really feels good!

serena: **I enjoy** sharing my blessings with others *a lot*. When I give to other people I feel so happy and special inside. It really amazes me that some kids get so excited that they start to cry because they've had a chance to meet me. One time, I got to bring a very excited college student on *Good Morning, America* with me. She was the winner of the Doublemint Aces for Campus Excellence program that Venus and I were involved with. College

"It really amazes me that some kids get so excited that they start to cry because they've had a chance to meet me."

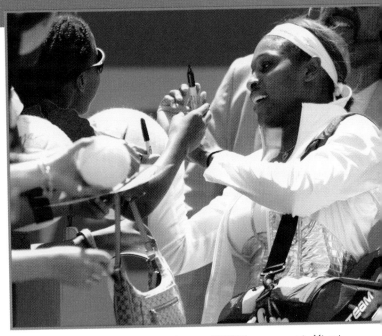

Serena signs autographs at the 2004 NASDAQ tournament in Miami.

students who were doing well in school and making a positive contribution to their communities were eligible to apply. They wrote essays or sent in videos describing their work and why they did it. Venus and I got to review all the essays and decide on a grand prize winner. We also got to select fifty $1000 winners. The grand prize winner won $10,000 in scholarship money and got to come on TV with me, which was a whole lot of fun! Then came the really fun part: She got $100 more each and every time Venus and I hit an ace—which we try to do as often as possible! In 2003, we hit about six hundred aces! All in all we raised an extra $60,000. So next time you see us serve one past an opponent, know that some amazing student just earned more money for college! Venus and I also help raise money in some of the communities where we play. The Family Circle tennis tournament is held in Charleston, South Carolina. Over the years I have helped local charities raise over $100,000 for different scholarship funds, helped community organizations to get books and comput-

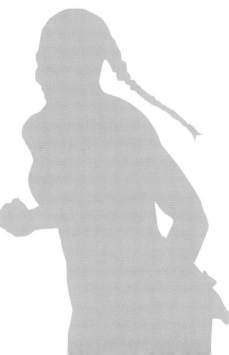

"You don't have to be rich or famous to share your blessings with others."

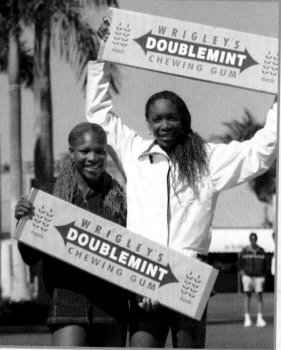

Venus and Serena worked with Wrigley's Doublemint, one of their sponsors, to support college students.

ers for a school library, and helped kids get involved in sports. Venus raises money for scholarships for kids in Charleston who are studying design and minority women who want to start their own businesses.

I have also gotten involved in several health charities. One of my friends, Linda Long, lost her mom to a disease called ovarian cancer, which I learned makes a lot of women very sick. I wanted to help her raise money so that more research can be conducted to help stop this disease, so I got involved with her foundation called "Players That Care." Other tennis pros participated, too— like Billie Jean King, who is still being generous and helping people out all these years later. I also played an exhibition tournament to raise money for the Massey Cancer Treatment Center at Virginia Commonwealth University.

VENUS: On top of the serious activities we do to help others, we also do smaller, fun kinds of things, like autographing tennis racquets and sneakers that we donate to organizations, who give them away. We also help different groups raise money by giving them items that they then auction off for cash—like the outfits we wear, for instance. Some of them can't be bought in a store, so people will always know that the person who's

"Sharing your money, time, and talents with others makes you feel great on the inside."

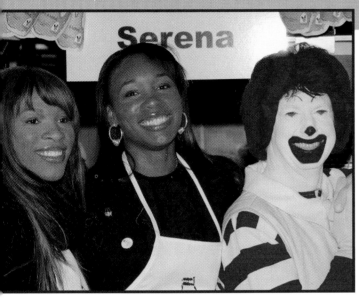

Venus and Serena help their sponsor, McDonald's, raise money for the Ronald McDonald House.

wearing it got it from us by contributing to a good cause. It's amazing to me that my dresses are worth a lot of money to people. I'm glad to give them away if it can help somebody else.

You don't have to be rich or famous to share your blessings with others. No matter what your circumstances are in life, there is someone who has fewer material possessions and opportunities or worse health than you do. Sharing your money, time, and talents with others makes you feel great on the inside. Even if you're feeling down, you learn how fortunate you really are and how much you have to offer. It takes the attention off your problems and makes you feel good that you have something that helps someone else. You find out that even though we appear to be very different on the outside, we all have much in common—the need for love, acceptance, and to know that someone cares for us. Helping others doesn't just improve their lives, it makes you a better person.

MAKE A DIFFERENCE AT HOME!

*Y*ou might be surprised by how good it feels when you contribute not only to your household but also to your community. Surprisingly, even small things can make a big difference.

Clean up after yourself and your environment! Be sure to recycle bottles, plastics, and paper when discarding trash. Don't litter.

Keep your bedroom clean and pick up after yourself in your home's common areas. Complete your weekly chores with a great attitude and no lip!

Volunteer

- at a soup kitchen feeding homeless people
- at an animal shelter
- at a hospital children's ward. Read to young kids who are sick and cooped up in bed or simply hold babies in need of comfort.
- at a nursing home. This can be especially rewarding if your grandparents are deceased or if there aren't any older people in your life.
- to tutor another kid at school in a subject that you're good at
- at a church, temple, or mosque. Offer to babysit the younger kids during services.
- to be a "Mother's or Father's helper" for a family in your neighborhood (especially one with a new baby!)
- with a church that delivers meals to older people who are sick or shut in at home
- to pick up litter blowing in your neighborhood and around your school
- to rake leaves, shovel snow, and sweep the stoop of an elderly neighbor

Do something nice for someone and don't tell them it was you. Just let the warm feeling glow inside you all day.

THE OWL FOUNDATION—
THAT'S WHOOOO!

Our mother founded the Oracene Williams Learning (OWL) Foundation to support kids whose families don't have a lot of money to have better educational opportunities in life. The foundation "adopts" schools, then raises money, and provides them with the funds they need to run special, educational programs. One year they even bought over $50,000 in computer equipment for some schools near where we live.

We're really proud of our mom's work and support it by visiting the kids and helping them with their homework. We help her raise money for the OWL Foundation by playing in an exhibition tennis tournament every year. People buy tickets to come see us play and the OWL Foundation gets all the money. It's always fun to play in front of a crowd. But it's even more fun to play in a sold-out stadium when you know that people bought their seats to help somebody else live a better life.

1/06